I0790488

Fitness:
Through the Eyes
of the Heart

Fitness: Through the Eyes of the Heart

George A. James

Copyright © 2021 by George A. James.

Library of Congress Control Number: 2021921115
ISBN: Hardcover   978-1-6641-1042-7
                 Softcover   978-1-6641-1041-0
                 eBook   978-1-6641-1043-4

All rights reserved. No part of this book may be reproduced or transmitted in any form or by any means, electronic or mechanical, including photocopying, recording, or by any information storage and retrieval system, without permission in writing from the copyright owner.

Any people depicted in stock imagery provided by Getty Images are models, and such images are being used for illustrative purposes only. Certain stock imagery © Getty Images.

Print information available on the last page.

Rev. date: 02/18/2022

To order additional copies of this book, contact:
Xlibris
844-714-8691
www.Xlibris.com
Orders@Xlibris.com
834606

Whatever your hand finds to do, do it with your might;
for there is no activity, planning, knowledge,
or wisdom in the grave where you are going.
(Ecclesiastes 9:10, NKJV)

Take delight in the LORD,
and he will give you the desires of your heart.
(Psalm 37:4, NIV)

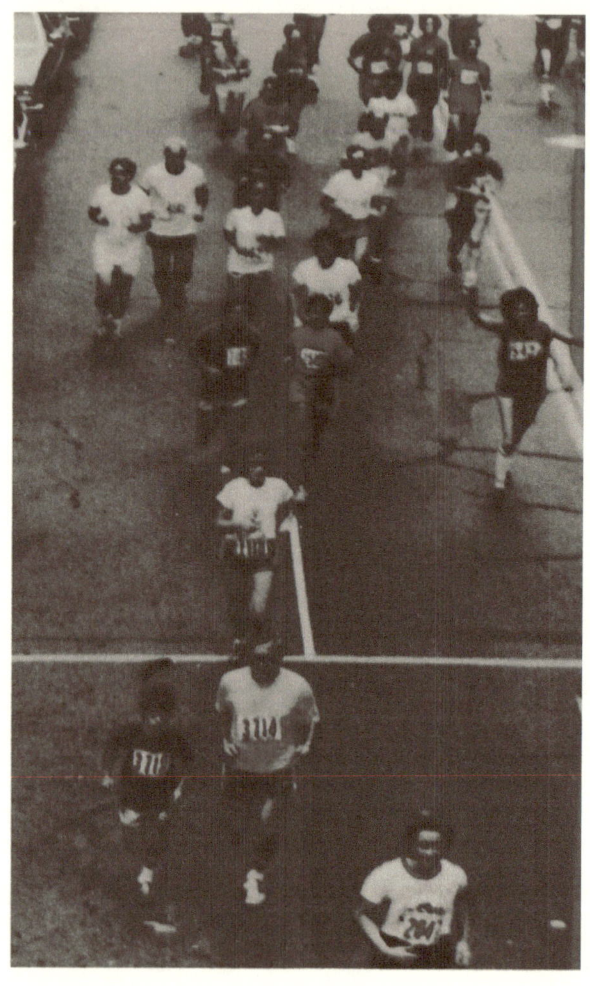

George James and Harry James crossing the finish line,
City of Pittsburgh, Great Race

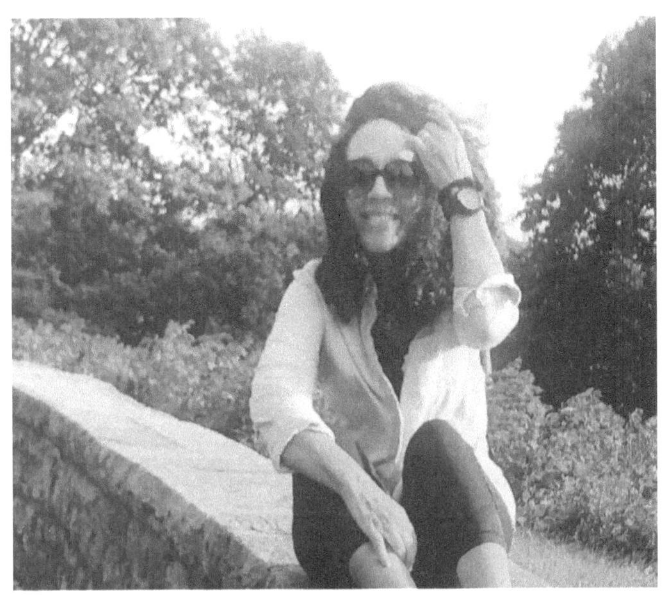

Carol, Dream Girl

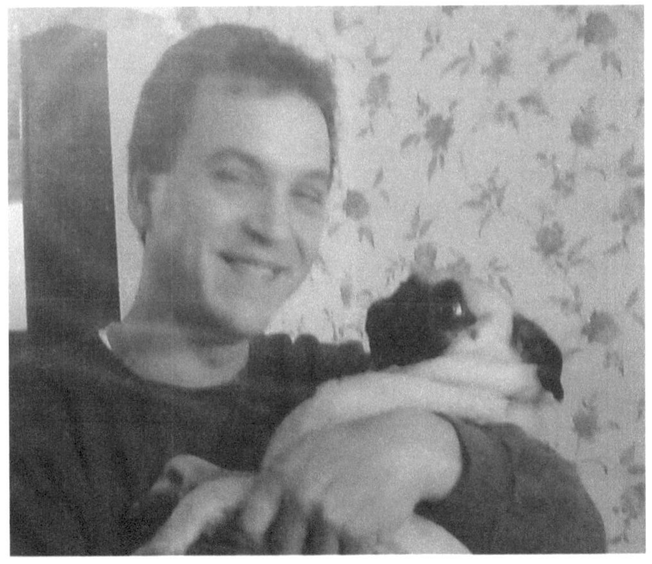

In Memoriam
Michael Aristocles James
July 20, 2020

Contents

INTRODUCTION

SOME YEARS AGO, a powerlifter went to visit a cardiologist. After being directed to the proper room, he carried his muscular five-feet, seven-inch frame down the hall where he would wait patiently for an experiment. The cardiologist soon entered, and the two exchanged warm greetings. Then the cardiologist began to prep his tools: a supine bicycle ergometer, nuclear camera, electrocardiogram, and computer. As he prepared his tools, he did so in an excitedly gleeful manner. After all, he was going to prove a point to the powerlifter—teach him a lesson. Himself a marathon runner, he had only other marathon runners as his subjects. His hypothesis was that the heart of a marathon runner would convincingly outperform that of a powerlifter. The cardiologist was ready. He gave his instructions, thinking to himself, *I've got something to prove to you today*. The procedure began. Twenty millicuries of technetium 99m was injected into the veins of the powerlifter. This substance is a radioactive tracer that attaches to red blood cells. The computer monitor, via radio-angiography, conveyed the systole and diastole action of the powerlifter's heart. What was of particular interest to the cardiologist was the left ventricle. This region of the heart is the most muscular, and it pumps blood to the entire body. With each beat of the heart, a percentage of blood leaves the left ventricle. This is known as ejection fraction, an important factor in determining the strength and vitality of the heart.

The intensity of the bicycle ergometer increased at consecutive intervals throughout the stress test. It began at 900 kg meter/min and climbed to 1,100 kg meter/min and then 1,300 kg meter/min. Each time the heart rate increased, so did the ejection fraction. It started around 79 percent and finished at 96 percent, with the powerlifter's heart rate climbing as high as 160 beats per minute toward the end of the test. What specifically was revealed? First, the blood flow to the powerlifter's heart via the coronary arteries was smooth-flowing—no obstructions. The cardiologist confessed that the powerlifter's heart, in regard to ejection fraction, had outperformed every marathon runner he had ever observed. Basically, the left ventricle of the powerlifter contracted to the extent that nearly every bit of blood was pushed out. It then relaxed and was able to fill up again for the next beat. Ejection fraction is very significant. It measures the amount of blood leaving the heart with each contraction. In this, the heart's squeezing ability can be determined. Recall also that this test included resistance. The resistance climbed significantly from beginning to end. Marathon runners often do not consider resistance training to be a significant component of their athletic performance. Powerlifters, on the other hand, are accustomed to plenty of resistance. The dear cardiologist appeared to neglect this critical point. The powerlifter outperformed the marathon subjects because they simply were not strong enough for the workload.

There are, however, other variables to take into account. Max VO_2, stroke volume, and heart rate are other forms of measuring the viability of the heart muscle. When the powerlifter compared max VO_2 to the marathon runners, he fell short of their mark. The average marathon runner has a VO_2 max of 75 ml of oxygen used by each kilogram of body weight per minute. Our powerlifter for this example had a VO_2 max of 55 ml. Max VO_2 uptake deals with the body's ability to utilize oxygen. This is the efficiency in getting oxygen to working muscles. This is the area where runners and aerobic enthusiasts excel. Interestingly, though, Dr. Mike Stone of Appalachian State University found that Olympic-style weight lifting of nearly five weeks of consistent training elevated max VO_2 by an average of 3 ml/kg/min in various subjects. Also, consider this. Are running, walking, cycling, and swimming the only way to train the heart muscle effectively? Fitness proponents advocate for at least three thirty-minute sessions per week of nonstop aerobic activity. If we do not receive this dosage, we are then shortchanging our fitness experience. Is this notion true? What did we learn from the example of the powerlifter and cardiologist? Whether one is running a marathon or lifting heavy iron, the heart muscle is still working and responding to the activity. How the heart muscle responds to various forms of exercise may be different, but it is nevertheless significant to all exercise. Is it more important to have a high VO_2 max or a high squat total with superb ejection fraction? Well, where does your perspective reside, and why? What are your fitness goals? Are you a powerlifter or a marathon runner? Did the powerlifter have a weak heart because his max VO_2

was 55 ml of O_2 for each kilogram of body weight per minute and most marathon runners have a VO_2 max of 75 ml of O_2 for each kilogram of body weight per minute? Of course not. His heart was trained differently and worked very well for him. Training specificity is the key difference between a powerlifter and a marathon runner. The important point here is that the heart is always working and responding to various kinds of stress. No matter what the activity, its role is always significant, and it responds accordingly. However, it is wise for anyone to be well-rounded in their approach to fitness as this may lead to reduction in injury, but the principle of specificity will dictate that some areas are sacrificed for a singular goal. Hopefully, in attaining a specific goal, a strong foundation of overall fitness has been firmly established.

CHAPTER 1

The Mystique of the Heart

DOWN THROUGH THE ages, poets, philosophers, and the Bible revere the wisdom, power, and faithful character of the heart, and through it, the impossible becomes possible. Ancient cultures believed the heart had a special role in relating to our emotions and character. Intrigue and fascination with the heart run through history. In the Old Testament book of Proverbs 4:23 (NLT), we read, "Guard your heart above all else, for it determines the course of your life," and in 23:7 (NKJV), we have, "For as he thinks in his heart, so is he." The wisdom of Job adds in chapter 38 and verse 36, "Who hath put wisdom in the inward parts? Or who hath given understanding to the heart?" (KJV). The New Testament also adds in Luke 5:22 (KJV), "What reason ye in your hearts?" Chinese medicine and yogic traditions perceive the heart to have both physical and spiritual components. In an ancient Chinese dictionary, it depicts how the heart and brain connect. In Japanese, *shinzu* describes the heart as an organ acting as a pump while *kokoro* relates to the heart's thinking ability. The multitalented Blaise Pascal commented, "We know the truth not only by reason, but also by the heart." Dr. Candace Pert, who authored *Molecules of Emotion*, has found a very curious relationship with the brain and the rest of the body. Pert explains that the brain communicates with the entirety of the body. This is accomplished through neuropeptides, which are commonly found in the brain but seem to be active everywhere in the body. Basically, the neuropeptides or peptides, which are amino acid chains, diffuse from one location of the body and attach to receptors of cells. All our cells have receptors that enable them to receive information and communication. In doing this, they give the cells messages on what the body needs to do. For instance, the body may need more rest, or it may need time for digestion after a large meal. Extremely fascinating, neuropeptides also are released from the brain during various emotions expressed by an individual. The heart responds to emotional changes as well. In essence, the whole human organism communicates in this fashion. The brain is not the only place that holds wisdom. Rather, an innate wisdom is found throughout the organism.

Similarly, other researchers have commented on the powerful neurological connection between the heart and brain. From the late 1970s and early 1980s, a field known as neurocardiology has been emerging. It considers the nervous system as well as the heart. Interestingly, thanks to the research of Dr. J. Andrew Armour of Dalhousie University in Halifax, Canada, we have come to learn the heart contains its own neural network, similar to that of the brain. The research depicts this aspect of the heart as containing neurons (which the heart has at least forty thousand of), neurotransmitters, proteins, and various cells. It appears the heart can act independent of the brain as it contains its own little brain with its own intuitive sense and reasoning capabilities. It also communicates with the brain. When the heart beats, neural messages are sent to the brain via the vagus nerve, which has parasympathetic afferent nerve fibers that send messages from heart to brain. The spinal column is significant here too in this process. The sympathetic afferent nerves use it in their communication from heart to brain. Specifically, the areas of the brain that are primarily affected are the medulla, amygdala, cerebral cortex, and frontal lobes.

The amygdala identifies with human emotion and the memories of various emotional experiences. Another portion of the brain the heart communicates with is the medulla, which has a neural influence on breathing and heart rate. The cerebral cortex governs our capacity to think critically and imaginatively while the frontal lobes decide what to do and what are the appropriate actions for a given situation.

Paul Pearsall, another researcher, adds similar insight in his book *The Heart's Code*. Each cell throughout the body receives biochemical nutrients from the heart. In this process of pumping and circulation, various forms of energy and information are also received by the cells. In this process, the heart, in essence, is communicating with the entire body. It communicates to the rest of the body through cells on how to function and work and what is needed at a given moment so our bodies are able to survive. This sounds deep and difficult to comprehend, and it is. The complexity of the human organism is undeniable, and the human heart may lead all other facets of the organism in its intricacy.

Cells are comprised of a membrane known as the cell wall, the nucleus that has our genetic blueprint, and a cytoplasm that maintains the structural integrity. The cells of the heart are similar to other organs and tissues in this way. There is something that makes the heart cells unique though. Heart cells pulsate. Other bodily cells do not. Skeletal muscle tends to weaken with age. Cardiac muscle does not weaken unless it has a disease. No other organ produces greater magnetic energy in the human organism than the heart. Poetry has rhythm, and so does the heart. Much of the finest poetry has been written in iambic pentameter, a steady beat or rhythm of words that simulates that of the heart. Likewise, there have been fascinating studies with the relationship of music and the heart. Music with seventy to eighty tones per minute coincides with the beating of the human heart, having a soothing effect on the human organism. Certain music beats similarly to the human heart, and certain styles do not. Classical music tends to have a calming or soothing effect on heart rate and brain chemistry while rock and roll music, for the most part, has an opposite effect. There was an interesting experiment conducted back in the 1970s. Some may be familiar with it. Dorothy Retallack used two sets of plants and exposed them to two very different styles of music. One group of plants was exposed to continuous rock music, and the other grew in the presence of placid-sounding devotional music. In roughly ten days, the plants growing near the continuous rock music began to grow away from the music. These plants would also wither and die soon after. The plants growing near the devotional music thrived and, interestingly, grew in a direction toward this style of music.

Australian doctor John Diamond has also investigated the fascinating effects of music on the human body. In his studies, he considered what is referred to as the "stopped anapestic rhythm" of rock and roll music. Bands that are considered in this category include the Doors, Eagles, Elton John, Rolling Stones, Stevie Wonder, and Janis Joplin. There are many others too. An electronic strain gauge was utilized while listening to this style of rock. Results of the experiment demonstrated that more than 90 percent of the participants lost muscle strength while listening to this style of rock and roll music. There were over a hundred participants. It gets even more interesting. Diamond observed a phenomenon known as "switching." A rearrangement of the alpha waves of the brain's hemispheres occurs that is similar to schizophrenics and babies. Included in his research was the loudness of music. *Any* music played at extremely high decibels resulted in muscle loss as well.

In an unborn fetus, the heart forms and starts beating before the brain even develops. Just three weeks after conception, the heart is beating, and the mother-to-be may not even realize it. During the course of our lifetime, it beats approximately one hundred thousand times a day. That means it beats about forty million times a year. The heart is capable of pumping two gallons of blood per minute or over a hundred gallons an hour. This is accomplished through a vascular system that is roughly sixty thousand miles long. Indeed, this is an organ that has captivated us spiritually, poetically, and from a physiological aspect as well.

From a physiological standpoint, cardiac muscle is similar to skeletal muscle but also different. Its striations resemble that of the skeletal muscle. The heart cells, however, interconnect in such a way that the stimulation of one heart cell causes a chain reaction affecting all.

CHAPTER 2

Heart Physiology

THIS EXTRAORDINARY FIST-SIZED organ beats roughly seventy times per minute. An adult heart may beat more than one hundred thousand times during the course of a full day. Along with this, nearly eight thousand liters of blood are pumped during the day. It is always working, beating, and does not rest. During an average human life span, the heart may contract up to two billion times or more. Four chambers comprise the heart muscle. We have the right and left atriums, which make up the upper chambers, and right and left ventricles comprising the lower. The ventricles are larger and more muscular than the atria, with the left being the largest segment of the heart. It receives blood from the left atrium and then pumps the blood through the aortic valve into the aorta. This artery then takes the oxygenated blood to the entire body. The right ventricle gets blood flow from the right atrium. It then pumps blood through the pulmonary valve, into the pulmonary trunk, and then to the lungs.

Together, the right and left atrium are the atria. These are slight in comparison to the more muscular ventricles. The superior and inferior venae cavae bring blood from the entire body to the right atrium. The left atrium is smaller than the right atrium. The pulmonary veins deliver oxygenated blood via the lungs to the left atrium. We can break this down further by saying the heart is essentially two pumps—the right and left heart pump. Each side has two jobs to perform. The right gets blood from all parts of the body and pumps it to the lungs. This is referred to as pulmonary circulation. In turn, the left side of the heart receives its blood from the lungs. The blood is oxygenated at this point. From here, the left side pumps blood into the aorta for delivery to the entire body. This we know as systemic circulation. Through the entire process of the cardiovascular system, nutrients and oxygen move through the body to where they are needed most. Wastes are removed in helping to maintain a healthy environment for the body. Blood carries oxygen from the lungs to the bodily tissues to be metabolized. The primary substance of this metabolism is carbon dioxide. The carbon dioxide then goes through the lungs to be eliminated from the body.

As mentioned above, the heart has four chambers. These chambers are affected by four valves. The atrioventricular valves are comprised of the tricuspid and mitral valves. They lie between the ventricles and atria. The mitral valve has two flaps while the tricuspid has three. Heart valves are responsible for the sound a beating heart creates. With a stethoscope, one is able to hear a two-beat sound of the heart. The closing of the atrioventricular valves causes this first sound. Closing of the semilunar valves, which are the pulmonary and aortic valves, causes sound number two of the heartbeat. These valves prevent backflow of blood. After the ventricles pump blood out, it is these semilunar valves that prevent the blood from coming back into the ventricles.

More specifically, the aortic valve is between the ventricle and aorta. The aorta is the primary artery that takes oxygenated blood out into the body. Because of the aortic valve's close tie to the aorta, it is stronger than the pulmonary valve. The pulmonary valve distinguishes the ventricle and pulmonary artery. This artery takes blood from the heart to the lungs.

Veins, Arteries, and Capillaries

The heart receives blood from the body by two large veins—the superior and inferior venae cavae. The superior vena cava takes blood from the upper body to the right atrium while the inferior vena cava comes from the lower body up through the diaphragm, sending blood into the right atrium. Also, the right and left brachiocephalic veins form the superior vena cava. They, themselves, are formed from even smaller veins from the head, neck, and arm region. The most prominent artery in the body is the aorta. It has an elastic quality about it that allows it to open wider and close comfortably. This recoiling of the aorta is for the pressure that is created by the blood flow. This helps enable blood pressure between beats. The aorta has a distinct shape with several sections. These segments include the ascending aorta, arch of the aorta, and the descending aorta. Each of these parts forms into smaller branches, which takes blood to the tissues of the body. So the veins transport blood to the heart while the arteries take blood away from the heart to the rest of the body. Capillaries are yet another key component in the cardiorespiratory system. They are very tiny blood vessels that measure in diameter from five to ten microns. Thus, this means they are a size red blood cells need to get into a single-file line to pass through. Capillaries deliver blood from arteries to the veins. They are prevalent in tissues and organs that have a high rate of metabolic activity, such as skeletal muscle and kidneys. Exchanging gases, by-products, and nutrients from the blood to the bodily tissue cells is the critical mission of capillaries. (Connective tissue, which consists of the ligaments and tendons, has little capillary saturation in comparison.) This occurs through the thin walls of the capillaries by the process of diffusion. The illustrations below depict the heart, veins, arteries, capillaries, and other significant characteristics.

Vessels of the Heart

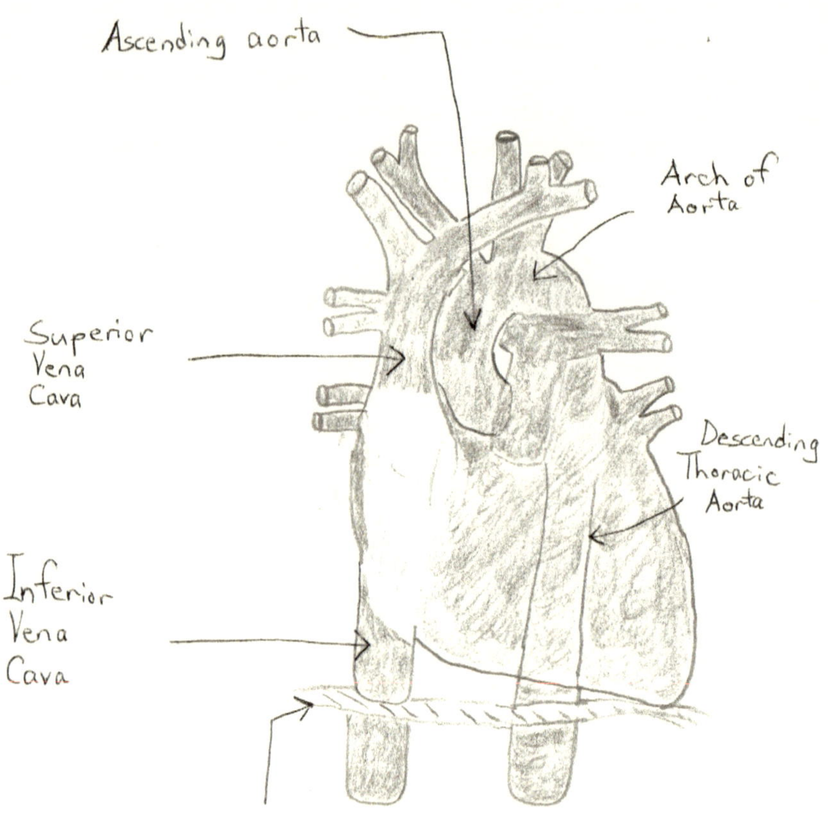

Fibrous Diaphragm
This portion of the diaphragm is intersected by the inferior vena cava.

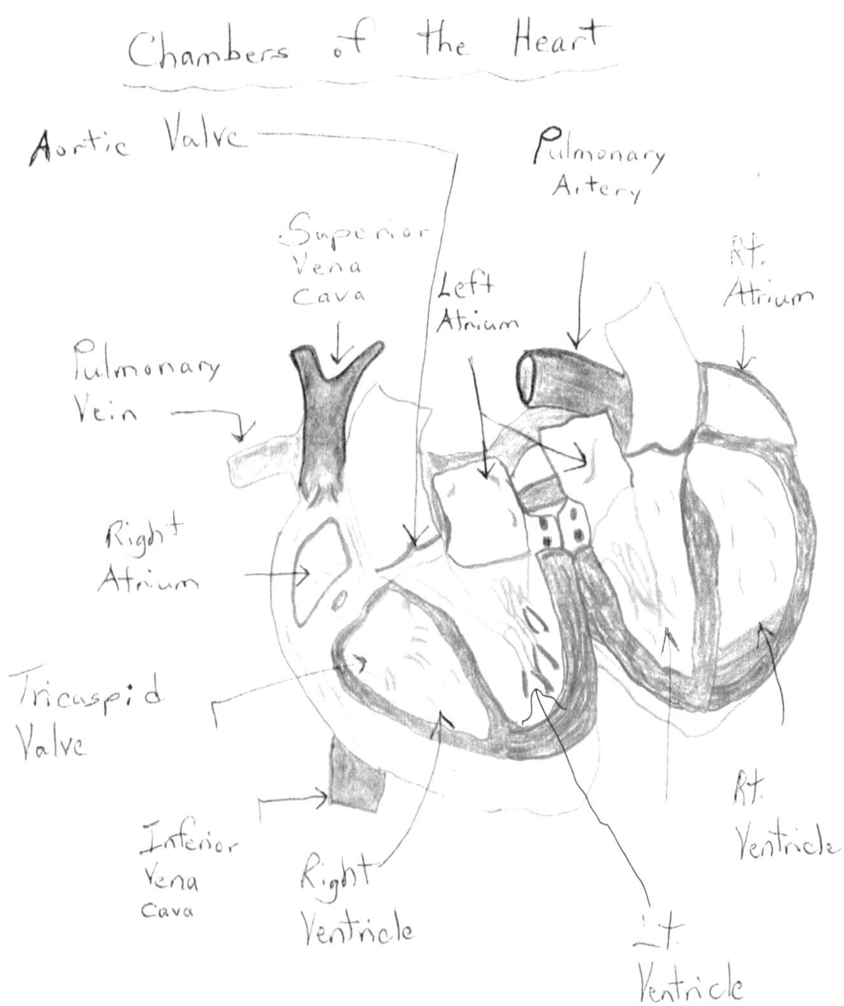

Internal Structure of the Heart Opened

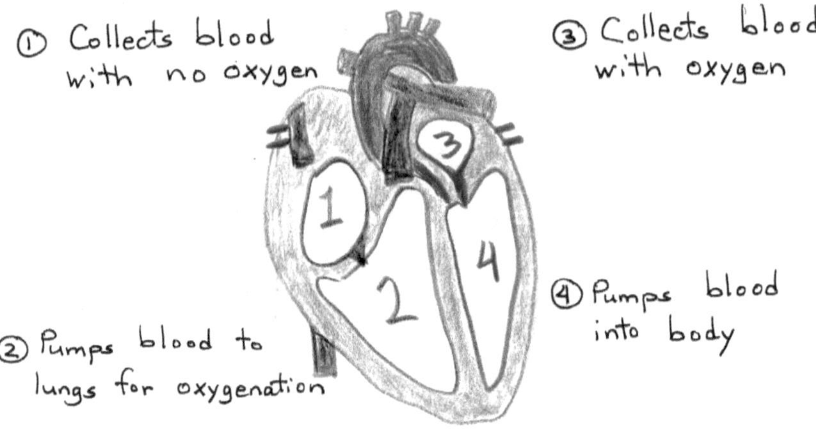

Depiction
of
Cardiac Cycle
① Collects blood with no oxygen
③ Collects blood with oxygen
② Pumps blood to lungs for oxygenation
④ Pumps blood into body
1
2
3
4

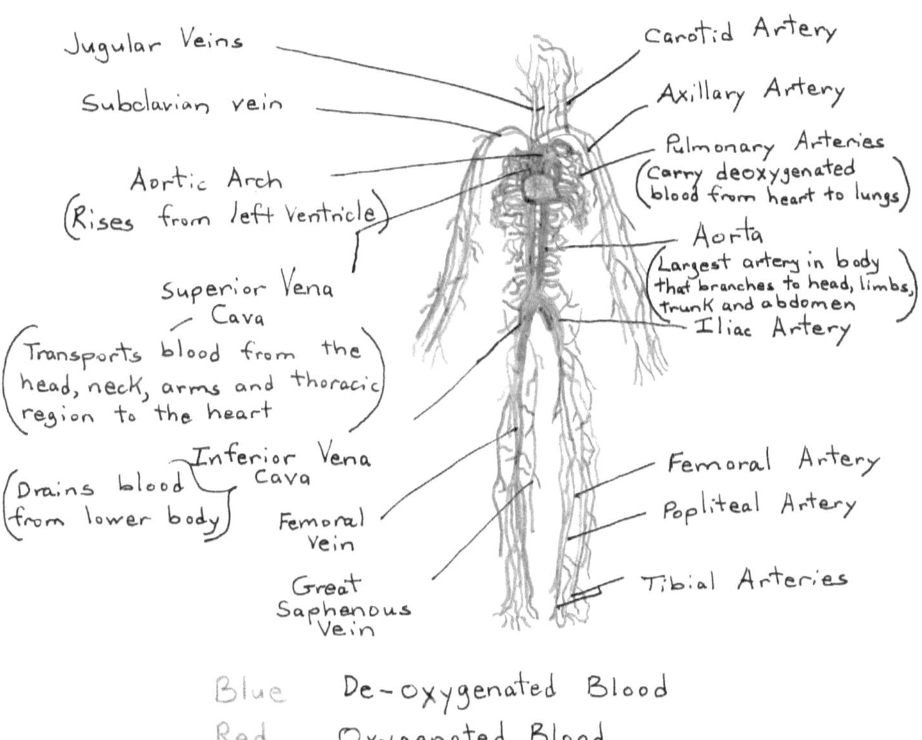

A Depiction of the Circulatory System
Jugular Veins
Subclavian vein
Aortic Arch
(Rises from left Ventricle)
Superior Vena Cava
(Transports blood from the head, neck, arms and thoracic region to the heart)
Inferior Vena Cava
(Drains blood from lower body)
Femoral Vein
Great Saphenous Vein
Carotid Artery
Axillary Artery
Pulmonary Arteries
(Carry deoxygenated blood from heart to lungs)
Aorta
(Largest artery in body that branches to head, limbs, trunk and abdomen)
Iliac Artery
Femoral Artery
Popliteal Artery
Tibial Arteries
Blue   De-oxygenated Blood
Red   Oxygenated Blood

A depiction of the circulatory system at a microscopic level

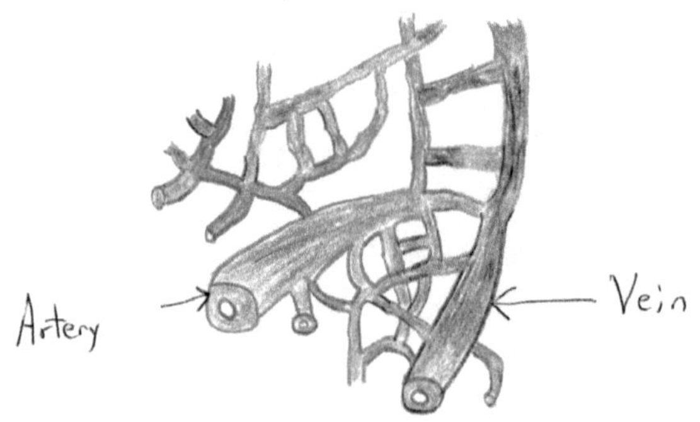

The arteries and veins become engaged by capillaries. Capillaries are between 8 to 10 microns and cannot be seen without a microscope. (a micron is 0.0001mm in diameter)

*An exchange of oxygen and nutrients occurs between the arterial and venous systems because of capillaries.

CHAPTER 3

The Heart's Response to Physical Activity

OUR HEART IS the key component in the cardiovascular system. Its pumping ability is impressive even for the moderately fit individual. Imagine the faucet of the kitchen sink in your home. When you turn it on to full capacity, it is a strong force of fluid. The maximum output of blood from the heart is greater than this force. It has to be. This force gets blood through an intricately designed vascular pathway leading to the working muscles. During prolonged continuous exercise like jogging, walking, swimming, and cycling, circulation increases to the muscular system. This is true for anaerobic activity too. As this is occurring, there is a contraction and relaxation of the muscles involved. This contracting and relaxing of the muscles send blood through the vessels and back into the heart. Cardiac output is the name given for the portion of blood pumped by the heart. It can be illustrated in this formula: Q = stroke volume × heart rate. Stroke volume and heart rate comprise cardiac output. Stroke volume is how much blood is ejected with each beat of the heart while heart rate is the speed in which the heart is beating. Two items can affect stroke volume. One is the amount of blood that can be pumped by the left ventricle after it fills up with blood. This can be referred to as the end-diastolic volume. The other pertains to the hormones of the sympathetic nervous system. These are epinephrine and norepinephrine. They create a more powerful ventricular contraction leading to greater systolic vacuity of the heart.

The Heart's Response to Aerobic Exercise

Generally, when one is performing aerobic exercise, cardiac output rises very quickly. This intensity levels off though if a comfortable level is maintained by the individual. Systolic blood pressure increases while performing at a moderate exercise level. After several minutes, it levels off to 140 to 160 mm Hg. The diastolic, or number on the bottom of the blood pressure reading, remains relatively constant with slight fluctuations. If exercise intensity continues to progress to higher levels, the systolic number may climb as high as 200 mm Hg depending on the fitness level of the individual. The diastolic number may rise only slightly from its pre-exercise number. If a maximal or near-maximal level is reached, cardiac output could climb to as much as four times the resting state. The cardiac output could then start from a level of 5 liters per minute and finish at 22 liters per minute. Stroke volume starts to climb right at the beginning of aerobic exercise. When an exercise participant reaches oxygen consumption of around 55 percent of their maximal oxygen uptake, it then levels off.

There are other considerations with the heart and aerobic exercise. Venous return is enhanced. This is the volume of blood coming back to the heart. Fibers of the heart begin to stretch in this process, which results in a more forceful contraction. This can be referred to as the *Frank-Starling mechanism*. It basically describes the contraction of the heart muscle having direct correlation with the lengthened muscle fibers. How one is able to utilize oxygen is another critical variable. Here we are dealing with oxygen uptake—how well the tissues of the body consume oxygen. This is often regarded as the most important standard in considering cardiopulmonary fitness. At rest, we can look at it this way: 3.5 ml of oxygen per kilogram of body weight per minute. How much oxygen needed by the working muscles is determined by three factors. These are the size of the muscles, their metabolic thoroughness, and the amount of work the muscles have to do. Recall earlier in the introduction, we looked at an example of a powerlifter in the office of the cardiologist. The powerlifter had a max VO_2 lower than the average marathon runner. This is not unusual. But realize that a person who is thin and lean will have an easier time for their muscle mass to consume oxygen than one who is thick and carrying much more muscle. Of course, the powerlifter outperformed the runners on the bike test because there was a resistance component to the test that steadily increased. Again, one is not necessarily better than the other. It is a matter of individuality and God-given muscle fiber type endowment. One should use and develop their muscles the best they can though for optimal health and wellness. Aerobic exercise that includes a great deal of large muscle mass correlates well with an increase in oxygen uptake and greater metabolic activity.

Of course, certain muscles could be more emphasized than others. In this case, the arterioles in the vicinity of the working muscles become dilated. This allows more blood flow and oxygen to the area. Simultaneous to this, the arterioles in other areas of the body will constrict, allowing less movement of blood to areas of the body that do not need as much blood and oxygen. While in a restful state, about 15 percent to 20 percent of cardiac output is utilized for the skeletal muscles, but with strenuous activity, this number can climb to 90 percent. Basically, being able to magnify the ability of the cardiovascular system will increase cardiac output for greater intensity in training and exercise.

Getting the most out of aerobic exercise requires one to focus on and be aware of their maximal oxygen uptake. A goal of trying to enhance this is integral for fitness goals in this area. Promoting cardiac output is again a key component here. Worth repeating, cardiac output is heart rate multiplied by stroke volume. Stroke volume is more significant in this equation. Stroke volume again is the amount of blood ejected with each beat of the heart. Ideally, one should see a lowering of heart rate with consistent aerobic training. This is an indication that the heart has become stronger and more efficient. A trained individual has a heart rate that increases more steadily than an untrained or sedentary person. Of course, we should recognize that overtraining can result in a higher resting heart rate for anyone. Balance and proper recovery is still an integral element for any form of fitness training.

Weight Training and the Heart

Many have the perspective that weight lifting is not a viable means for training the cardiovascular system. It is often believed that to train the heart muscle, one must get on a treadmill or take an aerobics class. The heart is always working though and will respond accordingly to all activity and challenges. In 2010, a fascinating observation was made at Appalachian State University. A comparison was made with a strength resistance exercise group and an aerobic exercise group. The resistance training group performed eight exercises along with three sets of ten repetitions for each, while the aerobic group performed thirty minutes of cycling. Variables observed included blood vessel widening, blood flow, and arterial stiffness. Vascular responses proved different for each group. Interestingly, there was greater blood flow to the limbs for the strength training group, although simultaneous to this, arterial stiffness increased with the strength training group. Contrasting this, the aerobic participants had greater arterial distensibility or less arterial stiffness. This may be surprising to some, but there was not an increase in blood flow to the limbs the way there was with the resistance group. It was noted by Dr. Collier and his team, who were overseeing this study, that the resistance group also had a greater drop in blood pressure. At the conclusion of this research, Dr. Collier and company recognize the significance of aerobic exercise in regard to promoting a healthy heart but are also staunch supporters of resistance exercise and its benefits to the cardiovascular system.

Anaerobic and aerobic exercise each elicits a response from the heart. Generally, weight training is a fast twitch muscle fiber activity, which correlates with anaerobic activity, with no or very little oxygen consumption. Aerobic training requires oxygen consumption and is usually accomplished over several minutes or longer. How resistance training is manipulated can alter its effect on the cardiovascular system. Lower weight and higher repetitions performed over a longer duration can have a similar effect as aerobic training would although to a lesser degree, but this is not true in every example. Intensity is also a significant component here. Cardiac output and stroke volume, for instance, may respond similarly to aerobic training if weight selection is low while repetitions are performed for a longer duration. This could mean the rep range may be between 15 and 25, or the reps could also be performed for more time under tension, which could result in greater muscle fiber recruitment.

If weight training is much heavier where great intra-abdominal pressure is needed, stroke volume may decrease. Heavier weight training can limit venous return and lower diastolic volume. Heart rate is a different matter. Heavy and light loads can both increase heart rate substantially. In fact, aerobic and resistance forms of exercise both stimulate the sympathetic nervous system to accelerate heart rate. Heavy weight training has no significant correlation with oxygen uptake though, unlike lighter loads, which will enhance the oxygen absorbed by the body and working muscles.

Some in the fitness world have suggested that weight training could cause the heart muscle to grow larger. In physiology, this is referred to as cardiac hypertrophy. There is indication that consistent aerobic training can cause this, however. The muscle fibers of the heart thicken, and protein synthesis can be enhanced. But in resistance training, for the most part, researchers in this area do not conclusively uphold this concept. Of course, there are always contrasting sides on any issue. There is some overlap between aerobic training and resistance training as pertaining to the heart. As mentioned earlier, most of these similarities are due to resistance training being done for a longer duration, for more repetitions, or with less rest between sets. Circuit training with resistance exercises can be one example where greater cardiac output can be developed. This is where exercises are done consecutively with little rest in between sets. High-repetition training where the reps exceed fifteen reps with a variety of exercises can be another strategy to induce greater cardiac output with weights. Peripheral heart action is similar to circuit training where an attempt is made to get blood flow through muscles of the entire body quickly with a wide range of exercises, but even here, it most likely does not match the cardiac output of regular intense running, cycling, or rowing activities. I say most likely because this depends upon the individual and their intensity level.

Exercising with weights and other forms of resistance also has an effect on blood pressure. A muscular contraction, which is maintained, compresses the peripheral arterioles, making blood flow more difficult. Naturally, this can cause an intense increase in blood pressure. Any form of weight training can spur this on, but the heavier the weight, the greater the response. For this reason, it is believed that individuals with existing high blood pressure and heart-related concerns should not engage in heavy weight training. Mark Rippetoe, author of *Starting Strength*, believes that individuals absent of preexisting conditions should be fine with heavy lifting. The pressure created with heavy lifting effects the cerebrospinal fluid in the cerebral ventricles and the blood pressure in the cerebral vasculature. The increase of each neutralizes the pressure of the other. There is nothing innately dangerous about this wondrous design of the human body. In super training, the late Mel Siff does warn, however, that those with preexisting heart conditions do need to be cautious of heavy weight training. For the most part, strength training, even with heavy weights and done with logical progression, can be a viable exercise means for many people.

There is also an interesting consideration when comparing upper-body and lower-body exercises. Blood pressure increases more with upper-body exercise. The upper body has smaller muscle mass and vasculature than the lower body. Greater systolic pressure is then required to get blood moving to the working muscles of the upper body. This could pose a concern for individuals with a compromised cardiovascular system. A more suitable approach for these people would be to perform walking, cycling, jogging, and "step"-type exercising rather than movements requiring primarily the arms. For very healthy and fit people, without the concerns of high blood pressure and other abnormalities, a wide range of exercise selections can produce wonderful results in promoting a heart that can handle sudden high levels of stress, increased metabolism, more efficient resting heart rate, and an overall stronger body with greater development of all muscle fiber types.

CHAPTER 4

Which Is Better?

IS THERE A best way to train the heart muscle? Is aerobic training superior to all other forms of exercise? Are there multiple ways to build a strong heart muscle or only one? I recall in several of my exercise science classes in college, components of fitness were discussed. Usually, it was expressed that cardiovascular endurance was the most significant of these components. It was believed by most of my professors and textbooks that cardiovascular endurance should be the most prominent of the fitness components because it pertained, to a great extent, to the heart and circulation. The reasoning here is that heart disease is so incredibly prevalent in society, so we should make it more durable with improved circulation through longer aerobic activity. There are, however, other strategies in building a strong, healthy heart. Steady-state rhythmic activity may have specific benefits, but as usual, there is another perspective to the matter. The questions above are some that physiologists, doctors, athletes, educators, and exercise enthusiasts have been asking and pondering for quite a while. What does the heart say about it? Let us ask it.

Understand first that whatever activity one is endeavoring to take part in the heart is always involved. It cannot help but be involved. In the previous paragraph, "components of fitness" were mentioned. Besides cardiovascular endurance, there are four others that are usually mentioned too: muscular strength, muscular endurance, flexibility, and body composition. From a collegiate perspective, this is generally what we are taught and understand. Components of fitness are not just limited to these. For instance, strength can be defined as the ability to perform an all-out effort or a single maximum repetition. This is limit strength. Many leave the concept of strength as this only, but strength and all forms of physical training and movement are synonymous with one another. Starting strength is the capability for someone to recruit many muscle fibers in an instant. Explosive strength or power is another example of how strength can be expressed. Once movement is initiated, the muscle's ability to remain activated for a specific period of time pertains to explosive strength.

To truly comprehend fitness is to see that defining it is quite elaborate. Delving more deeply, we can see other components that are often overlooked. Agility is an important attribute in many sports as well as dance. It pertains to quick actions of the hands, feet, and body. It also deals with body control and stabilization. Agility and running a hundred-meter dash at top speed are most definitely not the same thing. An NFL running back with 4.6 speed in the forty-yard dash can be very effective using agility to weave his way through the line of scrimmage to find daylight even if his running speed is nowhere near world-class.

Static balance and dynamic balance are also significant fitness variables. Static balance is keeping the center of gravity in line with the base of support. Basically, this is pure stabilization. Examples would include holding a side plank or balancing on one foot. Dynamic balance is the ability to keep charge of the center of gravity during motion. Examples here could be the snatch (an Olympic lift) and diving off a diving board as the body is spinning and twirling in the air before it hits the water. Muscular endurance, which was mentioned above, is performing many repetitions consecutively despite reaching levels of fatigue. This component can be identified further—local muscular endurance. Where muscular endurance pertains to a specific sport or exercise pattern, local muscular endurance considers a specified muscle. These are similar, of course, but different as well. There is also speed endurance. Someone who sprints for two hundred meters and is able to maintain their top speed throughout is showcasing excellent speed endurance.

With all these components, there is overlap. Some may argue that some of these components of fitness are basically the same thing, but that is not true when we consider specificity in sport and training. The muscular and nervous systems do not respond exactly the same in powerlifting and Olympic-style weight lifting. One who is great in one of these sporting endeavors is seldom great in the other. They both require strength, however. Powerlifting requires more limit strength while Olympic weight lifting requires greater power. But an Olympic lifter with very little limit strength will not be very successful, and a powerlifter with little explosive power may not reach his or her full potential. Various components of fitness and abilities are intermingled throughout different sporting and athletic endeavors.

As mentioned above, cardiorespiratory endurance (I am using cardiovascular and cardiorespiratory endurance interchangeably, but it is important to note that cardiovascular refers to the heart, blood, and blood vessels while cardiorespiratory pertains to all this and the lungs and breathing too. Some sources are more precise in this matter while others are more liberal.), which considers how well one is able to carry oxygen to the muscles being exercised, was once considered the most prominent of all fitness areas. This component pertains to the heart and lungs, and for this reason, it is given greater acclaim by many compared to other fitness areas. Is this true? What should we consider as we reflect on this?

Always remember that our heart muscle is always working no matter the activity. In the introduction, we considered a true story of a powerlifter compared to marathon runners. Recall some of the details there. The cardiologist conducting the study assumed the ejection fraction of the powerlifter would be inferior to that of a typical marathon runner. That was not the case in this example, however. The ejection fraction for the powerlifter proved superior compared to that of the marathon runners. This was where the contraction of the left ventricle pushed out every bit of blood but then was able to relax and fill up again for the next contraction. Recall, this was observed through a bike test where resistance was steadily increased. This was the key component because the powerlifter was able to handle the workload, but the marathon runners struggled because they were not as physically strong. This is an example where a higher Max VO_2 did not make any difference in the performance of a test that required a healthy, strong heart but also strong skeletal muscle too. As mentioned earlier, training specificity was the most significant component here. The cardiologist conducting the test was apparently unable to see that the marathon runners would not be as strong as the powerlifter as the testing continued with a higher-resistance workload. There is yet another interesting point for consideration. One who performs well in distance running will not necessarily perform as well in long-duration biking, swimming, or in an aerobics class. Why? Cardiovascular fitness is not just about exercising specific muscles for thirty, forty-five, or sixty minutes. All movement and exercise has a neurological aspect too. Cycling and running for instance are two separate activities where muscle pattern recruitment is quite different. One who is an elite 10K runner is not going to jump into the Tour de France and be elite in this event as well. The 10K runner may have a very low resting heart rate, comfortable blood pressure, and a high on the max VO_2 chart, but the movement pattern of running and cycling is very different, thus creating very different neurological input into the muscles for each sport. Both athletes may be very fit, but sport specificity matters too. We improve based upon specific adaptations to sport and activity.

In essence, this is referring to specificity in physical training. The marathon runners did have some advantages over the powerlifter, but the powerlifter had certain advantages too. Powerlifting requires a powerful effort over a short period of time. In this example, the heart actually works very hard in this brief episode. Heart attacks often occur because an individual cannot handle sudden intense stress. Long-distance running, even if it is done for miles at a time, does not create a heart attack-proof individual. Realize that what we are considering right now is long running that is done at a comfortable pace for long distances with little variation. Limited endurance training does not necessarily make one prone to heart attacks. They occur because of a quick or unexpected change in intensity. A very fast change in emotional status can also be a contributing factor. In essence, an abrupt rise in energy requirements is too much for the heart to handle, and a heart attack ensues because the heart cannot be supported by enough oxygen as there is a dramatic increase in workload.

This is not to say that long-duration steady-state activity has no bearing. Some in the fitness industry are advocating that steady-state aerobic activity is useless and a waste of time. All activities and exercise intensities have their place. The heart and lungs become more efficient with consistent aerobic training. A lower resting heart rate can result. Stroke volume may also be enhanced, and working muscles receive greater oxygen. The items above can fall under the term, eccentric cardiac hypertrophy. This is a specific type of cardiovascular adaptation. With this type of training only, something is given up though. Endurance may increase, but the ability to handle very stressful episodes in an instant begins to evaporate. There is another type of cardiac adaptation, concentric cardiac hypertrophy. (This is also known as reserve capacity). Cardiac muscle is working at high intensities in this example where the heart is not stretched but increases in size and thickness. Here, the heart rate is much higher during exercise, so the chambers do not have the time to fill with blood. This is due to the high intensity and speed of movement in which exercise is performed for this cardiac adaptation. Also, losing the ability to handle an onslaught of stressful conditions can possibly make one more susceptible to a heart attack. It is important to recognize that both of the above types of training affect the heart and can have a positive influence. It is just that training in only one fitness method may not produce the most optimal results for overall health and well-being. Training all muscle fibers through a variety of methods builds a strong, healthy, and resilient body.

It is a matter of opinion and personal belief that allows one to say that one form of exercise is superior to another. Many have assumed that aerobic training is the most critical of all because of its relationship to cardiovascular development. In my college days, I recall a professor stating this. But what happens when an individual is much older and they can barely get out of a chair? Is cardiovascular endurance more important than strength and balance at this point? How often do you think Usain Bolt would run a mile or more in his training? If he would run long-distance more often than sprint work, do you think he would have been as great as he was? Absolutely not. Fitness may be expressed in a plethora of ways, and the most important exercises are the ones that help you reach your individual goals and not the preconceived ideas of someone else. It is wise to be well-rounded though especially when establishing a thorough foundation or in the training of young athletes. Here is something else to ponder. We have this term *cardiovascular exercise*. A popular perspective is that to train the cardiovascular system, we should perform aerobic activities such as an aerobics dance class, bike ten miles, or swim or run a hefty distance. The plain truth be told—all exercise engages the cardiovascular system. Consider weight training. Brutally intense weight training stimulates the heart to a great extent. The heart needs to get an enormous amount of blood to the muscles that are lifting and controlling an intense resistance. With the skeletal muscle tissue creating strong powerful contractions, much support and engagement is necessary from the cardiovascular system. This is very stressful to the heart, and it will become stronger because of it. The amazing heart is always working and adapting to the stress we endeavor to place on it. Fitness comprises many things, and the heart relates to all.

CHAPTER 5

More to the Story

A CONSTANT THEME IN exercise circles is that to develop a healthy heart, the exercise of choice should be a long-drawn-out aerobic activity. This, going hand in hand with a low-fat diet, will safeguard against fat gain that will adversely affect the heart muscle and those dreadful unwanted pounds. There are other prevailing ideologies present. The one above has been a hallmark for many years now, so further investigation is warranted.

Have you ever noticed the various programs built into exercise machines deemed suitable for cardiovascular health? I recall a few years ago someone telling me they were working in the fat-burning zone on the treadmill. What did she mean exactly? There are three macronutrients our bodies use for energy: proteins, carbohydrates, and fats. Depending on the activity or intensity, our bodies utilize these macronutrients in varying amounts. Even at rest, the body uses proteins, carbohydrates, and fats. Roughly 5 percent of protein is used for energy when the body is at rest, for instance. During light-intensity activity, the body may use in the vicinity of 8% of protein for energy. With a moderate level, it is about 5 percent again, and with a high or very high intensity, a very low 2 percent is required. This makes perfect sense, for protein is never the key macronutrient for energy, but rather it is ideal for rebuilding bodily tissues and aiding recovery. An interesting note, protein is derived from the Greek word *proteios*, which means primary or holding first place.

With the other two macronutrients, there is a very different story for what the body uses for energy. In a restful state or casual activity, carbohydrates encompass 35 percent of energy requirement, and fats 60 percent. Please take special note of this and think. Would any reasonably thinking human being choose just sitting around to rid their body of unwanted fat? Get real. There is more pertinent information to cover here, so pay attention. A light exercise session uses 70 percent carbohydrate and 15 percent fat. Moderate exercise levels use 40 percent carbohydrate and 55 percent fat. High-intensity levels derive nearly 95 percent of energy needs from carbohydrate and only 3 percent from fat.

A pause is needed at this juncture. In the second paragraph of this chapter, a brief example was shared from an individual who claimed she performed her aerobic exercise in the fat-burning zone. Take special note again with the paragraph just above. Here, we read that during moderate exercise, fat is the greatest energy expenditure. This is correct, and this is what the young lady mentioned was referring to. To lose body fat and to maintain a healthy heart, she was performing moderate-intensity aerobic exercise for long durations according to the guidelines on the machine she would use. She had swallowed the conventional wisdom on exercise to burn body fat hook, line, and sinker. And while it is true that the majority of fat is burned at this intensity level, she was making an incredible flaw. Allow me to explain.

For roughly 22 years now, I have been involved in the fitness industry. I was training people before I received my exercise science degree. Every year has been a little different though due to military obligations along the way, although one of my roles in the navy has been to oversee the fitness and body composition testing too. A consistent observation has remained. Too often, men and women spend thirty minutes, sixty minutes, or longer on a treadmill, bike, elliptical, and StairMaster in hopes of attaining a desired outcome. This desired outcome of losing that unwanted body fat and transforming the body into the epitome of health is never realized. The human organism is a marvelous design with built-in intelligence of adaptation to stressors. Many believe that the longer they sweat doing some type of aerobic exercise at a moderate intensity, the more body fat they will lose. This is not what usually happens. While it is true that the body burns mostly fat during long-duration moderate-intensity activity, this strategy also teaches the body to be efficient at storing fat. After an exercise session is when the true intricacy occurs. Adaptation is a key ingredient in physical training. Remember, in long-duration moderate-intensity exercise, the body will burn mostly fat, so what do you think it does when exercise ceases? It stores more fat because it innately knows it will use it for energy the next time a long-duration exercise bout is performed. A sweaty hour of aerobic exercise done consistently produces an increase in body fat.

The Significance of Cortisol

Understanding the hormone cortisol is another relevant topic here. Cortisol is a stress hormone that the body releases via the adrenal glands, which are located above the kidneys. Cortisol is part of the hormone family known as glucocorticoids. Its levels are generally highest in the morning and during physical exertion. It can aid the body in feeling energetic and alive, but elevated cortisol too often has its downside. Fat storage is a means of survival, and constant elevation of cortisol promotes fat storage. Too much stress means the body will create cortisol with abnormal regularity. This can result in a loss of muscle and an increase in body fat because the body is unable to heal itself. Nonstop long-duration exercise activity proves detrimental in attaining fitness and wellness goals. This too has a strong correlation with cortisol. Staying up late at night fumbling around with the television, computer, or phone activates the senses. Cortisol levels are elevated as the body thinks it's earlier in the day, and it is time for more work, so sleep becomes difficult as it takes longer to unwind from the light stimulation. People who lack sleep are generally fatter and unhealthier. Additional body fat is always burdensome on the body and the all-important heart.

Adaptation

There is another important reality to comprehend. Starting a new exercise program produces positive results for just about anyone. The body is shocked and surprised by this new stress and responds accordingly. It adapts to the stress by becoming more fit, enhancing cardiorespiratory endurance and other fitness components depending on the training. Later, perhaps weeks or months, no further benefits will result if the routine remains exactly the same. At some point, and this is different for everyone, a new exercise stimulus is needed to produce elevated fitness levels. Now those with gym memberships and fitness staff have probably observed that there are specific members who have been slaving away on a treadmill, bike, elliptical, rower, or StairMaster for a year or more, and their bodies never change. They needed a new training approach, and they never provided their bodies with something different. They kept up with the same monotony, and adaptation occurred months prior. The body fat remained the same or perhaps increased. Consider cortisol again. This stress hormone remains elevated for the duration of all this drawn-out activity. Let's put this together. Many individuals in American society are believing if they can stay on that treadmill for an hour or more, it will compensate for the unhealthy lifestyle they choose to have the rest of the time. Getting little sleep and going to bed after midnight raises cortisol levels. Couple this with long bouts of aerobic sessions throughout the week, and a very sad situation arises. Cortisol levels are being elevated virtually all day. Cortisol elevation plus cortisol elevation equals too much stress on the body and serious gains in body fat.

Something Sinister

Another point needs to be mentioned. Some appear to never lose fat and unwanted pounds despite long aerobic sessions. Others, on the other hand, do. Pounds are dropped in certain examples, but so is muscle. Losing muscle is never a good contributing factor for health and wellness. Someone may have lost considerable weight. They are getting compliments galore for a job well done. Something sinister has occurred in this process. Skeletal muscle tissue has atrophied. Fat has come off along with pounds, but so has precious muscle. This leaves the individual, although lighter, softer, flabbier, and weaker. This is often coupled with caloric restrictions. A decrease in calories along with long workouts results in a catabolic state. Catabolism is a breaking down of tissues. Long workouts require quality calories. Without wholesome and a reasonable amount of nutrients, the body will not be able to recover completely. A combination of endurance training and caloric restrictions over time will eat away at skeletal muscle tissue. When there is a lack of calories from quality fats and carbohydrates, the body will use amino acids for energy fuel. Although it is true that the branch chain amino acids can aid with energy, the primary purpose for all the amino acids is to be building blocks for protein. Metabolism is drastically affected in this approach. It slows down, and the weight that was lost usually comes back. It comes back because there is less muscle. Muscle ensures that the calories that are taken in further its growth and development. Even at rest, muscle uses more calories than fat. An unhealthy caloric restriction mixed with long-duration exercise cannot last forever. Besides being unhealthy, it is not natural.

CHAPTER 6

High-Intensity Training

A S WITH THE previous chapters, this chapter has several relatable topics. High-intensity training can mean different things to different people. When a powerlifter performs a maximum effort with heavy iron, this is one example of high intensity. Anything a sedentary individual does can be high-intensity for them. Track-and-field events performed at the elite level are very intense, and training intensity for these events should mimic this to a large extent. There are a vast array of ways that high-intensity exercise or movement can be expressed. In the fitness and exercise world, high-intensity training is usually expressed through interval training. Interval exercise has fast powerful bursts of movement mixed with slower recovery periods. Virtually all life is done in intervals. Think about someone racing to catch a train. They get to the train breathing heavily, and now they are able to take a break and calm their breathing down. Most sports are similar. There is an intense play that lasts only seconds. This is then followed by a break in the action. A high-intensity effort is resumed again, and the cycle continues. Consider someone out for a morning stroll, and there is a hill or two involved. After expending a lot more energy walking to the top, the heart muscle now begins to calm as a level plateau is reached, getting the individual back into a steady state of exercise. Thorough research has indicated that some of the best results for fitness and health are accomplished with interval training. This type of training is brief but effective. Interval work uses energy from the muscles and not fat stores in the body. With its innate intelligence, the body responds to the type of training we put it through. The body adapts and stores more energy in skeletal muscle tissue rather than additional body fat. Remember that with long endurance and moderate intensity, the body learns to store more fat because that is the primary energy fuel for this type of training. Interval training promotes the utilization of carbohydrates being used for fuel. Fat is then burned for energy after the workout is over.

A research study at Colorado State University revealed pertinent information. The exercise session observed was approximately twenty minutes in duration. Two-minute intervals mixed with a one-minute "easy" segment was the depth of the workout. A key question for this study was, "How long does the body burn fat after exercise—not just any exercise though but interval training?" This study concluded that fat burning continued for sixteen hours after the exercise session. In a restful state, the participants' fat oxidation climbed 62 percent. Harvard has done similar studies in this area too. Here, a comparison was made with long-endurance exercise with brief exercise sessions that consisted of short intense segments. It was determined that shorter exertion with intense bouts built a stronger healthier heart in comparison to drawn-out cardiovascular endurance routines. Dr. Seiler, in conjunction with the American College of Sports, had an interesting report regarding interval exercise. He observed two groups: one who ran for twenty consecutive steady-state minutes on a treadmill and the other who ran for two minutes that produced heavy breathing and then two minutes of rest and recovery. His conclusion in this study was that interval training results in greater improvements in cardiac output than steady-state aerobic exercise. Interval training had another important attribute. It is superior to steady-state aerobic training because the heart learns it must adjust quickly to variations in intensity. In Dr. Seiler's project, stroke volume for the interval trainees was also superior to steady-state participants. Stroke volume is the greatest amount of blood the heart is able to beat when under duress.

Interval training has a positive correlation with cholesterol levels too. Research out of Ireland has confirmed this as well as Dr. Al Sears and his Center for Health and Wellness in Florida. A six-week interval program resulted in lowered total cholesterol and an elevation in HDL. HDL stands for high-density lipoprotein. HDL is often referred to as "good cholesterol," but in actuality, it is a lipoprotein, which carries cholesterol via the blood from one part of the body to another. One of the duties of HDL is to send cholesterol to the liver. It gathers cholesterol from arterial walls and other peripheral regions of the body. In the liver, it is excreted along with the bile, a yellowish-brown liquid produced by the liver, and enables the digestion of fats in the small intestine.

The *Journal of Applied Physiology* has observed a positive relationship with interval training and testosterone. Men who do intervals have greater testosterone levels than those who do endurance training. The oldest men in the study who did interval training had the most profound results in testosterone elevation. Testosterone is a crucial hormone for men and women. It is critical for the maintenance of muscle, sex drive, bone strength, and emotional optimism and well-being.

The Interval and Fat Burning Connection

Fat has been a prevailing concern in regard to health and vitality. This includes a strong correlation with heart health. Visceral fat, the fat in the abdominal region, is considered quite dangerous because it surrounds vital organs such as the stomach, pancreas, small intestine, liver, and colon. Subcutaneous fat is found above skeletal muscle and not considered as deadly. What is of particular interest here is the heart, like other organs, can also be affected by visceral fat, hence the name "fatty heart." This scenario lends itself to cardiovascular disease and abnormalities associated with the heart. When fat is closer to the heart, it causes greater damage because of the inflammatory proteins released from fat. This also adversely affects the bloodstream. To determine the amount of fat near the heart, a CT scan is necessary. This is not an optimal approach though. It is expensive, and a CT scan exposes one to radiation. Generally, more fat throughout the body increases the chances that more surrounds the heart too. So a CT scan is not necessary unless required for a very specific situation. Skinfold calipers with a competent administrator, hydrostatic weighing, and the Bod Pod will suffice.

Thank God exercise plays a vital role in defeating the detrimental effects of fat. The type of exercise conducted is critical though. Angelo Tremblay is one of the first to provide research with high-intensity exercise and fat loss. In 1990, Tremblay, along with other exercise scientists from Laval University in Quebec, Canada, had been studying data comparing moderate-intensity to higher-intensity exercise sessions. Included in the data were 1,366 female and 1,257 male subjects. These individuals participated in either an endurance training regimen or a high-intensity interval training regimen. A significant difference was observed. The ones who trained with high-intensity intervals were leaner. Tremblay and his colleagues recognized that most believe the key to fat loss is long-duration steady-state exercise—getting into that fat-burning zone. This fat-burning zone is believed to be reached at twenty minutes of exercise at a moderate intensity level. Beyond this point, the body will continue to use fat as its primary source of energy, so training for longer than twenty minutes is the best strategy for ridding the body of fat pounds. This was the conventional wisdom and still is among many in the exercise industry. Yet Tremblay and his colleagues observed something very different. With an honest observation of their participants and data, long-duration steady-state exercise did not produce the most optimal results for body fat and weight loss.

Tremblay and crew attempted to get a closer look in 1994. They honed in on their own specific hands on study with twenty-seven men and women. The group was divided into two separate exercise categories. One group was the endurance training group while the other performed intervals. The endurance trainees cycled for thirty to forty-five minutes at a consistent pace for their routines. This was done for eighty sessions over twenty weeks. High-intensity trainees had more variety to their approach. They began with several weeks of cycling at a comfortable pace for thirty minutes. This provided them with a fitness base. At the fifth week, a transition into interval training occurred. The workouts were very intense but also very short—lasting about four minutes tops. Ultimately, the endurance group would train for five weeks longer than the interval group and have twenty more workouts and a much longer training session. Results proved quite fascinating, though, in shattering conventional wisdom. Body fat and weight loss were measured before and after. The interval group lost significant subcutaneous fat, which was measured with skinfold calipers. The reduction in the interval group was nine times the difference on average than the endurance group. Body weight for each group remained roughly the same. Interval trainees basically lost body fat and gained additional muscle. Endurance trainees lost little body fat if any and gained virtually no muscle with their physical training. This is indicative of the interval group enhancing their metabolic rate. What we are dealing with here is caloric expenditure. There are calories burned during exercise. Exercise that promotes caloric expenditure after the workout is the type that leads to the most optimal health. This is precisely what interval training does because of the additional muscle development that goes along with it. Both groups burned calories during exercise. Interval trainees had their basal metabolic rate enhanced, energy expenditure at rest. Training for the interval group went beyond the workout. Interval training bolstered a metabolic response after the workout. The long endurance training did not do this. The inability of long-endurance training to promote muscle development is a critical aspect to this.

Other important notes regarding this study should be mentioned. It was one of the first studies of its kind that challenged the mainstream wisdom that long-endurance exercise produced the best results in reducing body fat and altering body shape. Further, the endurance group continued their program five weeks longer than the interval group. Twenty weeks was allotted for the endurance group and fifteen for the interval group. They had more time to produce better results but did not. Interval trainers also had much shorter workouts—four minutes for the interval group and thirty to forty-five minutes for the endurance group. Duration did not matter. Intensity and effort did.

In the 1990s, other significant studies emerged. Another notable researcher was from Japan, Izumi Tabata. Dr. Tabata also examined short intense interval training against much longer aerobic exercise. His studies encompassed maximum short-duration efforts coupled with short recovery segments. Similar to the results of Tremblay and his colleagues, Tabata's research proved that interval training was superior to steady-state endurance sessions. Tabata's work is unique in that he would emphasize maximum intensity while the majority of interval training does not. Interval training does not have to be the best effort possible all the time. It should, however, be challenging.

Many other researchers have come to similar conclusions. Dr. Ethlyn Trapp and colleagues considered interval training for a sedentary group of women. It was a study conducted in 2008, and unlike the Tabata protocol, it did not require maximum intensity. This study had one group of women perform eight seconds of intense work on a stationary bike and then ease up for twelve seconds. They exercised for five minutes at a time initially but finished with twenty-minute workouts by the end of this program. Women in the second group cycled for ten to twenty minutes initially and worked up to forty-minute sessions of steady-state moderate intensity. There was a third group that did no exercise. Each group participated in the program over a fifteen-week duration. The exercise groups trained three days per week. At the conclusion of this period, the interval group had superior results. There was a reduction in the inches around the legs and abdominal area. This included a drop, on average, of more than five pounds of fat for the interval group. Steady-state exercisers actually gained one pound of fat. This was a slight increase over the group that did no exercise at all. Fascinating. There are some vital lessons to learn from this. First, longer exercise sessions do not necessarily produce better results. Quality and intensity are key elements and not duration. Merely mindlessly slaving away pedal after pedal or step after step time after time will not yield the bodily transformation one is trying to attain. Also, earlier, we read about how the body responds to exercise. A review is in order, but we will build upon this concept as well. Recall that with steady-state aerobic exercise, after about twenty minutes or so, fat is the primary fuel. One would think that the steady-state group in this example would certainly burn the most fat. What happens after the exercise session is of primary significance. The body, with its own innate wisdom, realizes it needs fat for energy. It adapts to the demands placed upon it. So it stores more fat for future endurance exercise sessions. Shorter workouts that have interval segments result in a different adaptation. Energy is utilized from the skeletal muscle tissue—the glycogen stores. The body then learns not to store additional fat because it does not need to. Quick bursts of energy are needed and not the energy requirement that comes from long drawn-out endurance sessions.

When someone performs endurance training at a moderate pace, only one type of muscle fiber type is used—type I, which is slow twitch. Training this way does not build a strong, powerful body. It does promote greater endurance and an efficient cardiovascular system. A sacrifice of the skeletal muscle tissue occurs however. Type II A and Type II B fibers should also be trained. These are fast-twitch fibers, and the training of them builds a more powerful and attractive-looking physique. This enhancement of muscle development positively impacts metabolism. A more resilient and injury-proof body is also created. For overall fitness and well-being, training all muscle fibers through various types of exercise modalities is needed.

This is an excellent characteristic of interval training—getting all muscle fiber types involved. Genetically, the amount of muscle fiber type is God-given. An individual may have a large percentage of slow-twitch fiber or a significant amount of type II B fiber for explosive activity. Anyone, though, can enhance the capacity of their muscle fibers through specific training. Research from the 1990s does challenge the notion that we are simply born one way, and there is nothing we can do about it (Abnerthy et al. 1990; reported in Wilmore and Costill, 1994). Observations have been made where muscle fiber-type transformation has occurred through training with one method over a long period of time. No matter the individual, however, it is wise to have a well-rounded fitness approach. Even the greatest of athletes have some diversity in their training— particularly in their younger days. This can aid in longevity for years to come. Tudor Bompa, a world-renowned educator in the area of periodization, has written extensively on exercise programs that are balanced and age-appropriate. One of his hallmark points regarding children and younger athletes is to stress multilateral development—an approach that emphasizes many components of fitness and sports skills development. Do not be offended, but many adults need a similar approach because they lacked proper exercise development in their youth.

A Closer Look at Interval Training and Fat Utilization

Earlier, comparisons were made with steady-state aerobic exercise and higher-intensity work such as interval training. In the fitness world, a plethora of individuals are misinformed regarding the concepts of "fat burning" and "carbohydrate burning." Interestingly, even in a state of merely lounging around, both fat and carbohydrate are needed. We may be resting, but we are still alive, so the body needs and requires energy to maintain being alive. For most people, roughly 60 percent fat and 40 percent carbohydrate are required for each calorie of energy expended in a restful or sedentary state. The human body is using approximately 1.5 calories or kilocalories a minute in a restful state (McArdle et al. 1991). The old concept that we must exercise for twenty minutes at low intensity to burn fat is a myth. We burn fat even at rest for heaven's sake. So it does not take exercising twenty minutes or more to begin using fat as energy. Is a restful state an effective means to burn calories though? Of course not, at 1.5 calories per minute.

From rest to 50 percent of someone's max VO_2, the human body uses fat for a large supply of the energy needed. Most who work out at a gym go on their favorite aerobic machine and train at a level somewhere in this vicinity. Classes provide a similar intensity or could provide a more difficult challenge depending on the class. Remember though at an easy to low exercise intensity level, fat is not the only macronutrient used. Carbohydrates are involved as well. There is a key item to remain mindful of here. At a feeble exercise intensity, fat and carbs are burned at a sluggish rate—about three to five calories a minute. As exercise intensity picks up, caloric expenditure may range from seven to nine calories a minute. It is also true that at higher intensities, a higher percentage of carbohydrate is used for energy as compared to fat. With this much information, it appears that longer, slower physical training is the best approach for burning fat, but not so fast. There is more to discuss. With greater intensity, there is greater caloric expenditure, which ultimately causes more fat to be burned. This occurs because of greater oxygen consumption as intensity of exercise escalates. For every liter of oxygen that is absorbed, five calories are used for energy. Thus, intensity of exercise is very significant for goals of burning calories and fat.

Let's look at this another way. Even though there is a greater percentage of carbohydrate employed for each calorie burned with increased intensity of exercise, the percentage of fat multiplied by total calories used equates to a greater amount of fat expended for energy. Studies by Stanforth in 1989, Ballor in 1990, and Kaminsky in 1993 would concur with this. This can be illustrated further with these following examples:

First, it is critical to note that converting milliliters (ml)/oxygen (O_2) per kg of body weight to liters allows for a simpler process.

Additionally, one liter of oxygen is equal to five calories burned.

Example 1

- Exercise duration is 30 minutes.
- Subject has a max VO$_2$ of 34 milliliters (ml) of oxygen (O$_2$) per kilogram of body weight per minute.
- Weight is 198 lbs. or 90 kg.
- Convert ml to liters (L).
  * 34ml of O$_2$ × 90 kg = 3,060 ml/1,000 = 3.06 or roughly 3.1 L
  * 50 percent of individual's max VO$_2$ = 1.55 L of O$_2$ per minute
  * 1.55 × 5.0 calories per minute × 30 minutes = 232.5 calories burned
  * In this moderate intensity multiply 50% by the calories burned. 50% is the calories burned from fat. (.50 x 232.5 = 116 calories from fat)

We will now look at the same individual exercising for the same duration at a higher intensity.

Example 2

- Exercise duration is 30 minutes
- Subject has a max VO$_2$ of 34 milliliters (ml) of oxygen (O$_2$) per kilogram of body weight per minute.
- Weight is 198 lbs. or 98 kg.
- Convert ml to liters (L)
  * 34 ml of O$_2$ × 90 kg = 3,060 ml/1,000 = 3.06 or roughly 3.1 L
  * 75 percent of individual's max VO$_2$ = 2.32 L of O$_2$ per minute
  * 2.32 × 5.0 calories per minute × 30 minutes = 348 calories burned
  * In this higher intensity example multiply 35% by the calories burned. 35% is the calories burned from fat. (.35 x 348 = 122 calories from fat)

Note: 75% is not high intensity. It would fall somewhere between moderate and high intensity.

In the two examples above, the individual performed an aerobic exercise for thirty minutes for each workout. The intensity in the first example was 50 percent of the individual's max VO$_2$ and 75 percent in the second example. Although the duration of exercise was the same, the caloric expenditure in the second example was much larger—348 compared to 232.5 calories burned. The key here is not duration but intensity. Higher intensity burns less fat as a fuel source and more carbohydrate. However, as noted, there was greater caloric expenditure with the higher-intensity workout, and ultimately, more fat is also used for fuel. Basically, as mentioned above, the smaller percentage of fat used for energy multiplied by the greater number of calories burned for energy equals a greater amount of fat that was burned. In the examples above the difference of calories from fat is not very large. Keep in mind that exercising with higher intensity produces greater results, and these results have a cumulative effect over weeks, months, and years of consistent training.

Summary and Additional Notes

The examples above are very straightforward and simple. First, the individual trained at 50 percent of their max VO_2 and then 75 percent. The higher intensity produces better overall results, but more specifically, at a higher intensity of training, a greater amount of fat is burned. It may not be possible for many to maintain a 75 percent or higher intensity for the duration of their training. This is not a problem, and this is where the beauty of interval training comes into play. With interval training very high levels of intensity may be reached. There can be a substantial EPOC (Excess Post-Exercise Oxygen Consumption) result from this. This enhances metabolic rate. There is some debate on how effective EPOC results are. Still, it is widely understood that higher intensity training has a greater effect than lower intensity training on caloric expenditure even in a state of rest after the workout. Also, the EPOC effect may be greater if the workout is done earlier in the day.

CHAPTER 7

Measuring the Heart

VARIOUS METHODS HAVE been used to consider how hard the heart is working or should be working to elicit the desired response during exercise and as a means to improve upon health and current performance levels. They are not perfectly accurate, but they are helpful. Dr. Gunnar Borg, professor emeritus of Stockholm University and widely acclaimed for measuring intensity of experience, has made a notable contribution in this area with his Borg scale of perceived exertion. This is usually referred to as the rating of perceived exertion or RPE. Dr. Borg first presented this concept in the 1960s. Since then, it has been used in the medical community and with fitness coaches to establish a baseline for intensity.

Borg's scale runs from 6 to 20. Six would be a sedentary state, perhaps watching a movie, playing a video game, or reading. Nineteen and 20 would be exercising at a speed in which one could only maintain for a short duration. It is our best effort or the best effort we can give as the end of the race nears and were pushing for the finish line. The numbers in between these correlate with various activities. Seven to 8 could simply be putting on a pair of shoes. Nine to 10 is still very light activity with easy chores around the house. Eleven to 12 is fairly light but with more movement like grocery shopping. Of course, this is still not enough to escalate breathing in most people. A hike or brisk walk takes most of us into a somewhat hard level of 13 to 14. Heart rate and breathing go up but not to the point of labored breathing. When the heart is pumping fast and talking becomes challenging, it is a hard level and considered 15 or 16 on the Borg scale. A solid run, bike ride, or swim can produce this level of intensity. Seventeen to 18 is very hard on the Borg scale. This level of intensity is just a little lower than a maximum effort or something very close to that. It is a level in which significant progress can be made if the training level can be performed here on a relatively consistent basis. It is not so intense as to induce overtraining, but it is enough intensity to elicit the proper stimulus for improved strength, speed, endurance, and conditioning.

Realize that the Borg scale is a general guideline. Everyone is different. What is a 12 for one person may be a 15 for someone else. Improved conditioning will alter these numbers over time too. This is how it should be. A two-mile jog feels like 17 on the Borg scale, but several months later, it becomes only a 13. This is improvement in conditioning and endurance. The heart does not need to work as hard as it once did for this activity. It has become more efficient in its delivery of blood to the working muscles. The athlete senses the difference.

There is another interesting point about the Borg scale. It is a simplified way to estimate heart rate. The numbers 6 through 20 all correspond with activity, and each number on the scale multiplied by 10 gives an estimated heart rate based on the activity and how one feels during the activity or exercise.

Simplifying the Borg Scale

A scale of 1 to 10 could be used in place of the 6 to 20. In many fitness circles, this is the approach. Generally, people relate more easily to a 1 to 10 scale. At one site I worked at in Washington, DC, all the trainers had clipboards with a 1 to 10 scale on the back. When a member would be performing on a treadmill or some other aerobic machine, the trainer would show them the scale on the clipboard, and the member would give a number based on how they felt. This gave the trainer an impression of how the member felt during the exercise, and adjustments would be made if and as needed. Although the 1 to 10 approach is more relatable, the Borg scale may still give a more accurate representation of the heart rate when multiplying each number by 10. To keep things short, sweet, and simple, a 1 to 10 scale works just fine.

220-Age?

A popular method that has been used through the years is 220-age. Supposedly, this estimates maximum heart rate. After subtracting, multiplying the maximum heart rate number by 60 percent and 75 percent gives an exercise intensity frame to work with. This method and its suggested exercise intensities can be observed in fitness literature, various aerobic machines, and on charts in educational facilities. Although this might be a reasonable approach for many to use, it is not accurate. Think for a moment. 220-age is concluding that maximum heart rate is attained by considering age only. Genetics, the size of the individual, and current fitness level and training approach are not taken into consideration. Plus, the 220-age would have us believe that everyone has a maximum heart rate that diminishes with age in precisely the same fixed amount.

A Forgotten History

220-age has an interesting history. Its originators did not propose it to be for the masses but rather for individuals battling through cardiovascular rehabilitation. Foundationally, this approach for estimating max heart rate was based on a limited number of subjects who had similar fitness levels and abilities. This makes it unsuitable to cover a large population with a variety of individuals and fitness levels. In one research article by Richard King, he makes mention of the fact that the formula can be off by twenty or more beats in predicting max heart rate on the high or low side. Despite its shortcomings and lack of scientific accuracy, it is used continuously in educational literature and perceived by many as an appropriate standard for finding max heart rate (Kolata 2003). Another formula that attempts to find max heart rate is $208 - 0.7 \times$ age. This proposal did consider a larger population base. Thousands of subjects were included with an age range from eighteen to eighty-one with male and female subjects. Although it proved closer to an accurate depiction for max heart rate, it was still flawed and found again to over- and underpredict max heart rate by a significant amount (Tanaka 2001). Dr. Fritz Hagerman, exercise physiologist and was involved with the development of US Olympic and world rowing teams from 1972 to 2012, has studied the topic of max heart rate for more than thirty years. He has observed the max heart rates of Olympic-caliber rowers through testing and training and found that any formula that predicts a max heart rate is pure nonsense.

Karvonen Formula

A popular heart rate formula that purported to solve the inaccuracies is known as the Karvonen formula. It has its origin from Dr. M. J. Karvonen, developer of cardiovascular epidemiology in Finland. Dr. Karvonen had a very distinguished career in physiology, which dates back to the 1950s. Perhaps his most notable contribution is the formula he devised to calculate an appropriate heart rate for physical training. Acquiring the maximum heart rate and resting heart rate are necessary components for the calculation. The calculation again begins with 220-age despite the fact that published research for 220-age does not exist. This formula delves more deeply in that it tries to find a proper heart rate training zone by using resting heart rate. An example of this formula is laid out below:

* 33 years old.
* Resting heart rate = 73.
* Individual is trying to train within 60 percent to 85 percent of max heart rate.

220 – 33 = 187 (187 is the predicted max heart rate)

187 – 73 (RHR) = 114

114 × 0.60 = 68.4 + 73 = 141.4 (heart rate, which is 60% of target heart rate zone)

Above, 60% of the predicted training zone for the heart rate has been identified. Below, 85% of the predicted training zone for the heart rate has been identified.

220 – 33 = 187 (187 is the predicted max heart rate)

187 – 73 (RHR) = 114

114 × 0.85 = 96.9 + 73 = 169.9 (heart rate, which is 85% of target heart rate zone)

The training heart rate zone then becomes 141 to 169 for this individual. The perception is that training the heart in this range will enhance the endurance and strength of the heart. Below 141 is deemed too light of an intensity, and training consistently over 169 could cause overtraining.

Although the Karvonen formula aims to be more accurate by finding a training zone by considering resting heart rate, there are still shortcomings. Again, the formula begins with 220-age, a prediction equation with virtually zero scientific validity and grave inaccuracies. In 2000, Dr. Karvonen was contacted by the *Journal of Exercise Physiologyonline*. He was asked if he published original research of the 220-age prediction equation for maximal heart rate. He clarified that he did not but recommended the work of Dr. Astrand be investigated. In September of 2000, *JEPonline* was able to discuss the matter with Dr. Astrand while he was in Albuquerque, New Mexico, receiving a lifetime achievement award from the American Society of Exercise Physiologists. He also acknowledged that the genesis of the 220-age approach did not derive from himself. In discussing this further with *JEPonline*, he went on to elaborate that the 220-age was similar to other research that was conducted in this area and therefore probably good enough for what it is purported to do. For instance, another prediction equation Astrand may be referring to is 216.6 – 0.84 (age), another prediction equation that has proven to be highly inaccurate. *JEPonline* traced back the 220-age to Fox et al. Though, further study by Tanaka reveals that Fox cannot claim credit for establishing this equation.

Fitness Gadgets

An assortment of items are available for helping to measure the quality of a workout, the intensity level of the heart during exercise, and the conditioning level of the heart. None are as full proof as how a real human actually feels. This, of course, requires training and a deep awareness of the body's capabilities and potential. To get the most accurate representation of max heart rate, a clinically based test would be the most appropriate means. Heart rate watches can be helpful, however. Here is a little information. One such gadget is the polar watch and strap. Wireless heart rate monitors originated back in 1977 by Polar Electro. They were used as a training tool by the national cross-country ski team of Finland. 1983 marked the evolutionary point where wireless heart rate monitors became accessible to the average fitness enthusiast. Wired heart rate monitors, accompanied with several sensors, are generally used in hospitals. The polar devices, with watch and strap that goes around the chest and upper back, have been used in collegiate exercise physiology classrooms for quite a few years now as they can measure heart rate for a current situation and for reference in collecting data for research or study purposes. They can be a handy fitness tool for anyone—from the fitness enthusiast to the elite athlete. A heart rate monitor is a gauge to training intensity. They help someone judge if they should go harder, back off, or simply stay right where they are. It is a tool that may be used with a host of fitness activities, including walking, running, cycling, in-line skating, cross-training, circuit training, and group fitness classes. Interestingly, a study published in 1995 from *Medicine, Exercise, Nutrition, and Health* acknowledges that people who are in tune to their heart, even without exercise, may have less anxiety, depression, and anger. So just being in tune to the heart with a monitor may yield a positive emotional health response.

Many exercise machines are accompanied with heart rate monitors. How a treadmill or elliptical detect the heart rate is not ideal. The handheld sensors on these machines can be overly sensitive to every movement of the body, creating numbers that can jump all over the place. On occasion, people have told me that their heart rate is quite high when using a certain elliptical or treadmill, but they feel fine as if they are not working that hard. Some were concerned and thought they should back off. They were also confused because they placed a certain amount of faith into using these types of machines as a reliable source to dictate their exercise progress and intensity. These monitors should not be relied on for 100 percent accuracy.

The accuracy of heart rate monitors has been validated through clinical studies. When comparing an electrocardiograph with a heart rate monitor with corresponding strap, the results indicate, on numerous occasions, that the two devices read heart rate nearly the same. So a watch and corresponding strap can provide a consistent and reliable means to monitor the heart during various activity and exercise. This can aid in training more strategically in attaining fitness goals.

Other devices have evolved to enhance and keep track of the fitness experience. They include the Apple Watch. A series of Apple watches began in 2015. It can monitor heart rate as well as other fitness features. The two current Apple models include the series 3, which began in 2017, and the series 5, which had its genesis in 2019. The series 3 has an optical heart sensor while the series 5 consists of both the optical heart sensor and an electrical heart sensor with ECG/EKG capability.

Another is the GPS watch, which has numerous models. Many of these are considered smartwatches, but they are often used for the purpose of monitoring fitness. Apple has created GPS models, but Garmin, Polar, and Timex have produced more GPS models.

Activity tracker of fitness tracker is an additional tool for the fitness enthusiast or athlete. Some have been created to monitor heartbeat. They are usually more geared toward counting the distance walked or run and counting calories as well as formulating caloric expenditure. Some models may also provide a graph of heart rate and sleep quality. They are, in essence, an advancement of older models of pedometers. Two names involved in the evolution of activity trackers include Fitbit Surge and Samsung Galaxy Fit Activity Tracker.

Pedometers have been a long-standing fitness tool for many. It counts steps by detecting motion primarily through the hands and hips. This device can be overly sensitive. Routine activity such as bending down to lift something off the floor and hitting a bump while driving on the road may be counted as part of its overall steps for the day. In the past, pedometers have been digital (Omron HJ-112) and mechanical devices. Today, pedometers have been integrated into an assortment of electronic implements such as music players, smartphones, mobile phones, and watches (activity trackers). Specific products that contain pedometer abilities are Apple iPhone, Apple Watch, Fitbit, Nokia products, Sony Ericsson (W710 Walkman Phone and W580 Walkman phone), Android, and Samsung Galaxy S5. The pedometer is just one of several applications for these products. Below is a picture of a recent model by Apple—Apple series 6 watch.

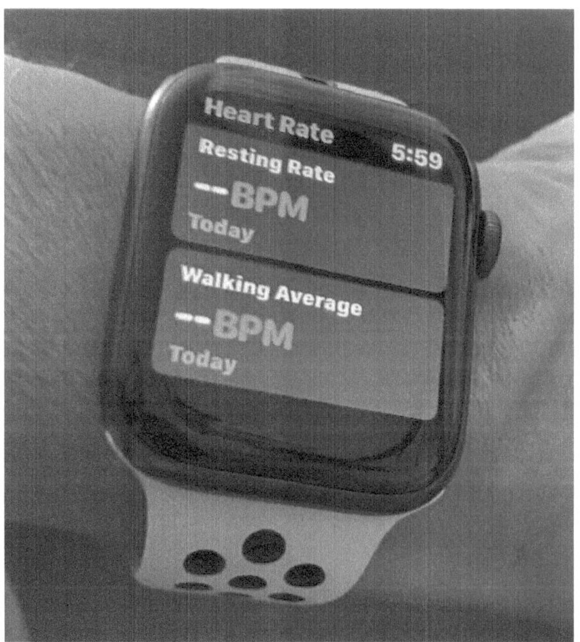

CHAPTER 8

Nutrition and the Heart

OUR HEALTH AND wellness and ability to move are products of the fuel we use for the body. This is often forgotten. A wide variety of nutritious foods can be beneficial for the heart. Good, wholesome nutrients can also keep us lean and mean. Healthy body composition is always less stressful for the heart. Heart-healthy foods may include the following:

1) Fish that are high in omega-3 fatty acid like salmon, trout, mackerel, herring, sardines, cod, and tuna. Eating fish like these has been shown to have a positive impact on blood pressure, blood triglycerides, and blood sugar level.

2) Flaxseeds and chia seeds also contain omega-3—a type known as alpha-linolenic acid. This provides cardiovascular benefits as well as blood sugar, digestive, and cognitive advantages too.

3) Walnuts are one of the healthiest nut selections. An integral part of their makeup includes micronutrients like magnesium, copper, and manganese. Research has indicated they can help in the fight against heart disease. One study observed a 16 percent lowering in cholesterol and a drop in diastolic blood pressure by 2–3 mm Hg. A separate study

of 365 participants showed similar results of diminished cholesterol levels. They may also drop levels of oxidative stress and inflammation.

4) Almonds are another super nut. They possess a quality list of vitamins and minerals. The heart-healthy monounsaturated fats and fiber are also attributes of almonds. One study considered forty-eight participants who ate 1.5 ounces of almonds daily for six weeks. The result was a loss of body fat for participants. A separate study done for four weeks revealed similar results. Almonds are also associated with reduced plaque and clear arteries.

5) Berries deliver phytonutrients and fiber. They also have special antioxidants called anthocyanins, which guard against inflammation and oxidative stress—two contributors of heart disease. Try some blueberries, strawberries, blackberries, and raspberries to name several.

6) Red, yellow, and orange vegetables are packed with carotenoids for a mighty heart. Some of these colorful vegetables are carrots, sweet potatoes, red peppers, tomatoes, and squash. Additionally, tomatoes contain lycopene—a plant pigment with helpful antioxidants. Lycopene diminishes oxidative damage and inflammation. These two items are detrimental to the heart. Research of lycopene has demonstrated that low levels make one more susceptible to heart attacks and stroke. It also frees up arteries from a surplus of plaque and cholesterol, so chances of heart disease are reduced. Carrots are a rich source of beta-carotene. This has a correlation with lowering heart disease and stroke. Sweet potatoes are packed with vitamins and minerals, including vitamins A, C, and E and potassium and calcium. Sweet potato skins are full of fiber too. Red bell peppers have the carotenoids beta-carotene and lutein. They also contain B complex, potassium, and fiber.

7) High-quality dark chocolate can be helpful to the heart. It is important to note that the chocolate choice should be about 70 percent cocoa. Chocolate also has antioxidants called flavonoids. Studies have demonstrated that there can be a 57 percent reduction in coronary heart disease and a 32 percent reduction of plaque in arteries from consuming chocolate on a consistent basis—perhaps five times per week.

8) Avocados contain monounsaturated fats. These are linked to a reduced risk of heart disease according to some research. Also, consuming an avocado a day in more than seventeen thousand subjects showed a less likelihood of metabolic syndrome. One avocado has roughly 975 mg of potassium—a mineral critical for heart health. About 5 grams of potassium can reduce blood pressure and minimize the danger of stroke.

9) Dark-green vegetables are a long-standing staple—most notably spinach, kale, and collard greens. They contain significant vitamins and minerals.

Vitamin K, for example, safeguards arteries and supports blood clotting. Greens contain dietary nitrates too. These maintain healthy blood pressure levels, create supple arteries, and enhance the cells that line the blood vessels. Consistent research with greens and lowered risk of heart disease has been maintained. Eight studies have observed the relationship between leafy green consumption and a lowered risk of heart disease, and a separate study with over twenty-nine thousand women observed a lowered risk for coronary heart disease.

10) Green tea has several healthy characteristics that can be helpful for the heart. It can be helpful in improving metabolic rate, burning fat, and improving insulin sensitivity. Polyphenols and catechins are natural ingredients in green tea that act like antioxidants. They prevent cell damage and inflammation—reducing inflammation is always heart-protective. Green tea may be beneficial to overall cholesterol levels as well. One study with green tea examined 1,367 people and determined healthier levels of blood pressure. Another study with green tea extract in the diet for three months showed healthier levels for blood pressure, triglycerides, and cholesterol.

11) Olive oil is very nutritious—possessing a rich source of antioxidants. It helps alleviate inflammation and decreases the risk of various diseases. Like other oils, it too is a quality source of monounsaturated fatty acids, which has a strong link to heart health. Studies on olive oil have shown a strong correlation with heart health. One study considered 7,216 individuals with a higher risk of heart disease. Olive oil consumption showed a 35 percent reduction in the risk of developing heart disease in this group. Another investigation demonstrated olive oil lowering the susceptibility of heart disease by 48 percent, and yet a larger study observed the positive effect of olive oil on lowering blood pressure.

12) Garlic has a long-standing history with good health—heart health included. Allicin, a natural ingredient in garlic, is a significant component of this. Garlic extract, taken in 600–1,500 mg doses for twenty-four weeks, demonstrated a positive effect on blood pressure. A review of thirty-nine studies on garlic indicated that its consumption showed promising results for those with high cholesterol levels. Still, other research illustrated garlic's ability to diminish platelet buildup—minimizing blood clots and stroke.

13) Whole grains are considered a heart-healthy food. Specific types include whole wheat, brown rice, oats, rye, barley, buckwheat, and quinoa. Numerous studies have revealed a correlation with whole grains and a healthier heart. Forty-five such studies were lumped together. In observing them closely, it was determined that three or more servings

of whole grains daily resulted in a lowering of heart disease risk by 22 percent. A separate analysis observed three servings of whole grains dropped systolic blood pressure by 6 mm Hg. This is enough to reduce stroke by 25 percent.

14) Beans have resistant starch. This type of starch resists digestion and is fermented by the good bacteria in the gut. Resistant starch can reduce the blood triglycerides. One study of sixteen participants found eating pinto beans can drop blood triglycerides and LDL cholesterol. An overview of twenty-six studies saw a correlation with consuming beans and legumes and a decrease in cholesterol. Eating beans on a regular basis has also been correlated with a drop in blood pressure and inflammation—two risk factors for heart disease. Other bean selections could include black and kidney beans. These are also good sources of fiber, B-complex, magnesium, calcium, and omega-3 fatty acids.

Supplements for Heart Health

One of the most popular heart health supplements is coenzyme Q10. It is most often referred to as CoQ10. The history of CoQ10 dates back to its discovery in 1953, compliments to Dr. Frederick Crane. He initially believed it was common to vitamin A. By 1957, he recognized it was something truly different as he located it in cow heart. About a year later, a biochemist, Karl Folkers, from the University of Texas along with a pharmaceutical company produced a means to make it more accessible. American researchers, for the most part, did not see its important health benefits at this time. The pharmaceutical company sold the groundwork for creating CoQ10 to Japanese scientists. So it was Japanese researchers of the late 1950s and 1960s who determined how valuable this could be for overall health—particularly pertaining to heart health. The Japanese began to discover that CoQ10 could aid in congestive heart failure. Western society lacked focus in nutrition and CoQ10 and adhered to open heart surgery and medical drugs instead. As research in CoQ10 advanced, it also became known that CoQ10 was and is a powerful antioxidant. These are various nutrients, vitamins, and minerals that protect the body against different forms of stress. Antioxidants are especially noted for fighting free radicals, which can cause an array of health issues: Alzheimer's, heart disease, cancer, and arthritis to name a few. Free radicals are defined as highly reactive molecules that do damage to protein bonds of an organism's tissues, DNA in the cells, and polyunsaturated fatty acids in the cells' membranes. CoQ10 protects cellular health and provides energy to vital organs.

Studies of CoQ10 in hospitals and universities are numerous. It is valuable for all vital organs and the immune system, but its correlation to heart health is most significant. CoQ10 has proven to have a rich history in its relationship to cardiovascular disease. Dr. Folkers, mentioned earlier, did not give up his studies of CoQ10. He and a different team provided a solid foundation with CoQ10 and its relationship to heart health as well. His team noted low levels of CoQ10 in individuals with heart disease. From the 1970s reaching into the early 2000s, there have been at least fifty studies considering the supplemental use of CoQ10. One very notable study was contrived by Dr. Folkers and Dr. Langsjoen. Their work started in 1985 and lasted until 1993. 424 individuals took CoQ10 and mainstream heart medication. The New York Heart Association functional scale was used to monitor patient progress. This scale rates heart disease from I to IV (from least serious to most serious). The results depicted a powerful outcome with CoQ10. Fifty-eight percent of the individuals improved to the next category, 28 percent advanced two categories toward better heart health, 1.2 percent had a three-category improvement, and 43 percent reduced or disposed of their medication altogether—a very impressive improvement.

Blood pressure has resulted in more comfortable numbers with CoQ10 supplementation. The *Journal of Human Hypertension* reported an interesting double-blind study. Here, there were two groups of individuals with hypertension. The study was conducted for an eight-week period with one group receiving a placebo and the other receiving CoQ10. The CoQ10 group reduced blood pressure significantly.

A study in *Molecular Aspects of Medicine* revealed interesting results. Individuals who were taking medical drugs for high blood pressure began to supplement with CoQ10. In time, more than 50 percent no longer needed their original prescription drug for high blood pressure. Another study at the University of Texas revealed similar results. In this study, one month of CoQ10 supplementation resulted in 51 percent no longer needing blood pressure medication.

Congestive heart failure is another abnormality. It can affect either the right or left side of the heart. Recall that the left side of the heart distributes oxygen-rich blood from the lungs to the entire body. The right side of the heart sends blood that is depleted of oxygen back to the lungs where the oxygen is replenished. With congestive heart failure, this process does not work so smoothly. If there is damage to the left side of the heart, the blood backs up into the lungs. This causes shortness of breath, a dry cough, and wheezing. The right side of the heart may also be damaged. Other problems result. Blood remains stagnant in the legs and liver. This leads to swollen feet, swollen ankles, swollen neck veins, pain inferior to the ribs, and fatigue. It has been found that low levels of CoQ10 have a high association with congestive heart failure. The mitochondria of the cells also appear to be affected.

Traditional medication may benefit congestive heart failure to a certain degree. The overall prognosis is not very positive. A five-year survival rate is only 50 percent. For many others, the survival rate is only a few months or maybe a couple of years. Once someone has congestive heart failure, there is usually little time remaining.

In its supplementation, CoQ10 has proven quite helpful to patients with congestive heart failure. One of the key aspects with CoQ10 is that it strengthens the heart cells. It can also promote a healthier-functioning heart. It has enhanced the lives and years for patients with a failing heart. One study confirmed in *The Doctor's Heart Cure* that CoQ10 cuts the average yearly death rate for heart failure by 33 percent.

CoQ10 has proven beneficial with other abnormalities. Angina pectoris or myocardial ischemia should also be mentioned. Nearly three million Americans suffer from this. It is a combination of high blood pressure and coronary artery disease, which cause the heart muscle to become deprived of oxygen. Several items may set off angina attacks. Exercise, emotional upheaval, and even digesting a heavy meal can trigger angina attacks. These attacks are critical because they can be a harbinger of a full-blown heart attack. CoQ10 is helpful once again. One example demonstrates this in a double-blind study—a study in which neither the doctor nor patients know who receives the placebo and who receives the supplement or medication. In this example, twelve individuals who took 150 mg of CoQ10 for four weeks displayed a 53 percent drop in their bouts with angina attacks compared to those who took the placebo. In addition, those who received the CoQ10 displayed greater output in their treadmill sessions.

Studies in Australia also proved fascinating with CoQ10 involved. One study used the hearts of young and old rats. The hearts were placed in a device so they could beat artificially. Great stress was applied to make the hearts beat to excessive levels—500 beats per minute for two hours. At the end of the test, the younger hearts regained 45 percent of their ability. Older hearts recaptured 17 percent of their capability. Then a second phase of the study was added with two new groups of rats. One group was given CoQ10 for a period of six weeks and the other a placebo. Unfortunately for the rats, they were liquidated, but their hearts were used in the same marathon-type test mentioned above. The results proved fascinating. Young rat hearts performed virtually the same whether or not they had taken CoQ10. The older rat hearts that had taken the CoQ10 supplement recovered equally as well as the younger ones.

This can relate to older adults who have to go through heart surgery. People over the age of seventy do not do very well in heart surgery. "Reperfusion injury" appears to be the primary problem. For the purpose of surgery, the heart needs to be stopped so an operation can be performed on it. Circulated blood is given to the body during the surgery by a heart-lung machine. At the conclusion of surgery, the heart is restarted. This is overwhelming though because the magnitude of oxygen causes free radical damage to the heart. Free radicals are unstable cells that steal electrons from other cells. Remember, CoQ10 is an antioxidant. Antioxidants neutralize free radicals. How can CoQ10 help the heart when it is stressed by the "reperfusion injury"—the stopping and then the restarting of the heart for the purpose of surgery?

Similar to the rat heart experiment, a group of cardiologists placed heart tissue in a mixture that included oxygen and glucose. An electric wave was administered through the mixture, which caused the heart tissue to beat. The strength of the beating heart tissue was then measured. Later, researchers stopped giving the heart tissue oxygen and glucose for an hour. This would be similar to an open heart surgery as mentioned above. Oxygen and glucose were again added. This would also cause free radical damage once again too. Younger heart muscle outperformed older heart muscle—70 percent to 49 percent recovery. The test was then performed again, but this time with the older heart muscles receiving CoQ10 for thirty minutes prior to testing. It was determined, once again, CoQ10 made a valuable difference in the older heart tissue's recovery. In fact, the older heart muscle exceeded that of the younger heart tissue by 2 percent on average. It should be recognized that the younger heart tissue did not receive the CoQ10 in this study, but CoQ10 can help older hearts regain their youthful vitality. CoQ10 has proven to be a valuable supplement for nearly everyone. It neutralizes free radicals. These can damage the heart and general health. Additional studies have taught that CoQ10 can limit problems with cholesterol and reduce the risk of heart attacks.

Other Heart Supplements to Consider

Nutritional supplements have proven to be beneficial for the heart. Our first line of defense should always be quality foods. In a busy stressful lifestyle, we can often miss getting enough of the important nutrients that are needed to thrive, not just survive. Supplements can aid in filling in the gaps.

Various studies have proven this to be the case. Twenty-two thousand Americans took part in a US Department of Agriculture study in the early 1990s. It was revealed that a meager 4 percent obtained their recommended daily allowance (RDA) of important vitamins and minerals. Interestingly, there are nutritionists who would claim that the (RDA) is not adequate. Later, a more recent study concluded with similar findings. It is believed that 91 percent of Americans do not eat enough fruits and vegetables, and 70 to 80 percent are deficient in getting appropriate levels of vitamins C and A. Our nutritional sources are not as nutritionally sound as they once were. Spinach, for example, has only a miniscule amount of the iron it had in 1948 due to the change in farming practices. Spinach is also a source for vitamin E—an important antioxidant for heart health too. It takes twenty-five cups of spinach to just receive the RDA requirement for spinach. Of course, there are other sources for spinach, but the point is that sometimes our food choices do not meet the body's needs for nutrient requirements. Zinc, an important mineral for the immune system and healthy hormonal balance, is another nutrient devoid in most diets. Sheri Leiberman, nutritionist and contributor to the ISSA's *Specialist in Performance Nutrition* course, talks about eating for survival and eating for optimal performance. Eating for survival is precisely that. It is surviving or just doing enough to get by. It does not consider individual stress for each person. Eating for optimal performance is getting the nutrients needed to thrive for all daily activities. It considers the daily challenges and to have energy and strength needed for all of them. This may require greater nutrient intake than the RDA and proper supplementation especially since most Americans have little variety in their food selections as well. Linus Pauling, Nobel laureate, also understood that all should strive to go beyond the recommended daily allowances for vitamins and minerals. He recognized that merely surviving is not thriving in a life of energy and zeal.

The paragraph above should be enough to realize that supplements are a wise investment for anyone striving for greater health—including heart health. Remain mindful though that a well-rounded diet with nourishing foods takes precedence. Supplements are second but still important for a variety of reasons. There are additional supplements that are superb for the heart. CoQ10 was discussed previously.

Heart-Healthy Nutrients

First, we will look at L-carnitine. It is similar to CoQ10 because of its energy-producing capabilities at the cellular level. Carnitine has been classified as a vitamin and an amino acid. It is neither, although it does contain characteristics of both. A more accurate depiction would be to define it as a short-chain carboxylic acid with nitrogen. It is also water-soluble like B vitamins. Carnitine transports long-chain fatty acids into the mitochondria of cells. This affords the human organism the opportunity to utilize this fat for energy. Carnitine keeps this cycle going—burning fat and producing energy. Consistent burning of fat promotes a healthy heart, liver, and skeletal muscles by reducing the risk of heart disease, diabetes, and high levels of triglycerides. Carnitine is present in areas of the body that require great amounts of energy such as the heart, brain, muscles, and testicles.

Numerous studies have demonstrated positive results on how L-carnitine promotes heart health. Arterial plaque reduction, lower-LDL cholesterol, and an increase in HDL cholesterol have all been associated with carnitine in more than twenty placebo-controlled studies.

Red meat and dairy are both optimal sources for L-carnitine. Vegetarians and those with dairy allergies and who are lactose intolerant should consider supplementation. Choose a natural L-carnitine supplement and not the synthetic D, L-carnitine. Those who eat red meat should choose grass-fed and organic meat sources as often as possible. How the animal was raised and treated while alive does make a difference in the quality of the meat and nutritional content. Five hundred milligrams of L-carnitine as a supplement is a reasonable level for health and vitality.

L-Arginine

L-arginine is another critical and helpful substance for heart health. Supplementing with L-arginine can be a much safer means to combat heart and circulatory problems than prescribed drugs. It is an amino acid that is an antecedent to nitric oxide. In the bloodstream, L-arginine becomes nitric oxide. Nitric oxide opens blood vessels that line the heart, allowing them to be supple and elastic. This is in contrast to arterial plaque, which creates rigidity and a restriction of blood flow.

Food sources for L-arginine include red meat, fish, chicken, beans, chocolate, nuts, and seeds. As a supplement, 500 milligrams is a sufficient daily dose. The L-arginine form is best. Besides its heart benefits, L-arginine is also supportive of skeletal muscle growth and development.

Vitamin E

Vitamin E, a fat-soluble vitamin, is another key factor for heart health. Like CoQ10, it is also an antioxidant. The *New England Journal of Medicine* has reported high marks for vitamin E and heart health. One of the reports observed eighty-seven thousand females for an eight-year span. A separate study observed forty thousand males. A segment of each group took 100 IU or more of vitamin E. Through the course of this period, it was determined that 41 percent of the women had a reduction in their risk for developing heart disease. Likewise, 37 percent of the men showed the same conclusion. A reduced risk for stroke and death rate was also indicated by those who took vitamin E as a supplement. Its ability to enhance blood circulation is one of its best attributes.

There are points about vitamin E that should be adhered too. Vitamin E appears naturally in foods as four tocopherols and four tocotrienols. Many of the vitamin E supplements contain only the alpha-tocopherol type. This can interfere with the absorption of the other components of vitamin E. Tocopherols and tocotrienols are found together in a variety of foods—meat, fish, oils, nuts, seeds, dark-green vegetables, and avocados.

A supplemental dose of 400 IU with 5 milligrams of tocopherols and tocotrienols together is a sound recommendation. Similar to CoQ10 and vitamin D, vitamin E is a fat-soluble vitamin. For best absorption, almond butter, olive oil, fish oil, or other healthy fat choices should be consumed along with a supplement of vitamin E.

Vitamin C

Vitamin C is probably the most popular antioxidant. It is noted for its immune defense and collagen formation among other things. It too has proven to have a strong correlation to cardiovascular disease. Low levels of C have been associated with stroke during a ten-year study of more than 2,400 male participants. It was revealed that vitamin C levels have more of an impact on getting a stroke than high blood pressure and body composition.

A study from the University of California revealed other interesting details. The study included several thousand men. Men with the highest intake of vitamin C demonstrated the least risk for dying of heart disease. Primarily, these were men who took vitamin C supplements. Those who took the daily recommended allowance through food exhibited virtually no protection against heart disease. The recommended daily allowance is only 60 milligrams. This is enough to prevent scurvy but not enough for optimal immunity and overall health. Vitamin C is a water-soluble vitamin, so it does leave the body very readily through exercise and other forms of stress.

Foods that have C include citrus fruits, strawberries, broccoli, dark-green vegetables, and bell peppers. Five hundred milligrams to 1,000 milligrams a day is a good recommendation for vitamin C intake. To help prevent viruses and colds, 3,000 to 5,000 milligrams may be necessary.

Homocysteine Levels

This is an area that has been misunderstood and neglected by nearly everyone. Homocysteine is a naturally occurring amino acid in the body. At a certain level, though, it is toxic and damaging to the body. High levels of homocysteine in the blood prevent proper dilation of blood vessels. This restricts blood flow and can lead to heart attack or stroke. It is generated during metabolism—producing energy for what the body needs to do. In biology terms, we can refer to this as an example of oxidation within the body. This process can be detrimental if it spreads and is unchecked. Antioxidants like vitamins C and E, carotenoids, and CoQ10 resolve this problem. In essence, there is a strong correlation with homocysteine and antioxidants. The antioxidants combat homocysteine from injuring tissues and from increasing to an extreme level. The level of homocysteine is an indication as to how healthy an individual actually is.

Homocysteine indicates optimal antioxidant levels in the body, but it also is indicative of cardiovascular health. A blood test can determine homocysteine levels. Less than 8 mmol/l is believed to be a healthy level. High levels of homocysteine will hurt arteries. It increases arterial plaque and causes platelets in blood to become stickier. The stickiness of platelets makes blood clot formation more prevalent. This magnifies the chance of a heart attack, stroke, or pulmonary embolism. Numerous studies have indicated a high correlation with elevated homocysteine and heart attacks as well as strokes. One such study was the Physician's Health Study. It indicated individuals with high homocysteine levels have a heart attack risk threefold that of other participants. Homocysteine proved more significant than cholesterol levels in causing heart attacks and strokes.

There are many causes for high homocysteine levels. A lack of B vitamins is one of them. The good news is this can be easily remedied. Key B vitamins to keep homocysteine in check include B2, B6, B12, and folate. These B vitamins subdue high homocysteine levels and return it to an appropriate amino acid level.

Meaningful doses of these vitamins are 25 milligrams for B2, 25 milligrams for B6, 500 micrograms for B12, and 800 micrograms for folate.

Interestingly, most have not heard of homocysteine. This includes patients who have suffered from, and are currently suffering from, heart and circulation ailments. There are no commercials advertising homocysteine-lowering drugs. Pharmaceutical companies pushing the sales of homocysteine-lowering drugs are nonexistent. Drugs are not needed for this. Al Sears, a cardiologist in Florida, uses vitamin supplementation for homocysteine, and it is effective. Drugs are not always the answer, and there are usually negative repercussions.

C-Reactive Protein and Heart Disease

This area provides another indicator for heart health. C-reactive protein (CRP) is released by the liver as the body undergoes stress of various sorts. CRP should not be found in the bloodstream. It could be a serious indication of heart health concerns. The *British Journal of Urology* reported on a correlation with CRP levels and heart attacks. CRP levels of nearly four hundred participants were observed. It was revealed that for CRP levels doubled the normal level, the possibility for a heart attack increased 150 percent.

The *New England Journal of Medicine* provided similar results in 1997. Twenty-two thousand men were observed for eight years. At the beginning of the study, all were free of heart disease, and blood samples were taken from each. During the eight-year span, fifty-four were compared with those who did not have a cardiovascular disease. It was determined that those with highest CRP levels had two times the risk for stroke and three times more likely for a heart attack. What is very interesting to note here is that the CRP levels were a predictor of this eight years prior when the blood samples were taken for all.

Studies have considered the CRP levels of women too. CRP can be a predictor of heart attacks for women. Brigham and Women's Hospital and Harvard Medical School conducted a joint study. They found women with high CRP in their blood were more than four times more likely to have a heart attack.

Everyone can benefit from knowing their CRP levels. C-reactive protein is measured in units. Very healthy people have a unit below one. Four units usually indicates signs of heart disease. A level near twenty indicates an individual is close to death. Physicians are able to test these levels as part of an annual examination or by special request. High CRP levels may also indicate additional health concerns like rheumatoid arthritis, rheumatic fever, cancer, tuberculosis, and pneumonia.

Insulin Related to Heart Disease

The correlation between insulin and heart disease has been overlooked by many in the health profession. The pancreas is the key organ when it comes to insulin. When carbohydrates are ingested, it controls glucose, a type of sugar, in the bloodstream by releasing insulin. Under optimal circumstances, cells absorb glucose from the blood due to the communication from insulin to do so. This gives the cells energy. When blood sugar levels are depleted from physical activity, the liver then frees stored glucose so a regular supply of energy is available.

There is a concern with insulin. It stimulates fat storage in the body and burns fat at a slow rate, causing fatigue. A condition of insulin resistance is currently a very significant topic. The cells do not take up adequate amounts of glucose. This puts additional stress on the pancreas to produce more insulin. There is a serious problem with this. The pancreas may stop producing insulin because it's too tired. Glucose levels then climb to high levels in the blood, causing someone to develop type 2 diabetes. This is also known as adult-onset diabetes.

There is a genetic component to this, but lifestyle choices are important too. Weight management needs to be considered. If someone allows themselves to gain a lot of weight and doesn't do anything about it, it will be very difficult for them to get back to a healthier weight later on. A sedentary lifestyle is usually the biggest culprit when unwanted weight gain occurs. Exercise helps the body metabolize insulin and glucose so unwanted weight gain may not occur. Food choices are equally significant. Simple carbohydrates like white bread, bagels, doughnuts, and Pop-Tarts should be avoided, or at least not be a main staple in anyone's diet. These are high-glycemic index foods. They elevate blood sugar in the body, causing the release of insulin—a fat storage hormone. Healthier food selections of quality protein sources and extra-virgin olive oil can combat this.

Insulin resistance is a blood sugar issue. It is, however, tied to other health abnormalities. High levels of triglycerides, cholesterol problems, high blood pressure, and also heart disease are all related to insulin resistance. Yes, heart disease is related to insulin resistance too. Many who have this problem struggle mightily with their weight. Excess body fat is a problem for diabetics, and it most certainly is a problem for the heart.

It is helpful to be aware of insulin levels. A blood test by a health-care provider can determine this. Normal insulin levels are considered to be between 7 and 17 mcU/mL. This is microunits per milliliter. A number above 17 mcU/mL has a strong correlation with diabetes, hypoglycemia, and obesity. It is important to mention that people with diabetes are sometime found to be in the lower range. A good goal would be to have a number below 10 mcU/mL. Healthy, lean athletic people have been known to have numbers at 7 mcU/mL or lower.

CHAPTER 9

Workouts, Training, and Fun

EXERCISES AND MOVEMENT are vast. A solid walk, jog, or run performed at a comfortable pace is a foundational approach for many. This is referred as a "steady state." On the RPE (rate of perceived exertion) scale, this would be a 5 on a scale from 1 to 10, or 50 percent of maximum heart rate. When exercise is begun, the heart rate elevates. The heart rate remains the same if the intensity levels off and remains constant. The intensity could be lower than a 5 on the RPE or higher. Our bodies adapt to stress rather quickly and are able to handle the load or pace placed on it. The steady-state pace is fine for establishing a fitness base for anyone who has been sedentary or inconsistent with exercise. Below are some possible scenarios:

1) Walk/jog for 30 to 45 minutes on Monday, Wednesday, and Friday.
2) Walk/jog for 15 to 30 minutes on each day Monday through Friday.
3) Jog/run for 30 to 45 minutes on Monday, Wednesday, and Friday.
4) Jog/run for 15 to 30 minutes on each day Monday through Friday.

A jog is just a little faster than a walk but still could be quite slow. A run is a little faster than a jog. In the run, the stride is opening up. The run is still performed at a steady-state pace, however. This will be different for each individual, but the pace should be comfortable.

Note: if you are currently only able to walk, that is fine. Still find ways to make it more challenging as your fitness improves by walking faster, using hand or ankle weights, walking backward and sideways, and trying some hills.

The time frame above may also be conducive to using exercise machines such as indoor bike, elliptical, treadmill, and StairMaster. Swimming or hiking can be other alternatives too. All these fitness endeavors can be done at a "steady state" or comfortable pace for the one doing the exercise. To reiterate a point from above, this approach is suitable for anyone who has not been exercising consistently, is new to exercise, or wishes to get back into a regular routine. This is not a wise exercise regimen for the long term. The body adapts quickly, and improvement on this type of regimen will wane after a relatively short period of time.

Below are pictures of some aerobic exercise choices that can be done with a steady-state training strategy:

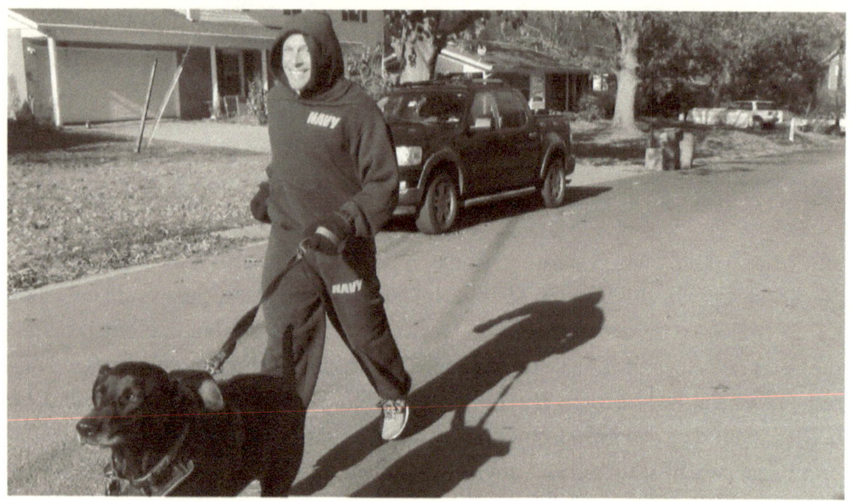

A comfortable run in the neighborhood with Gabriel Dimas

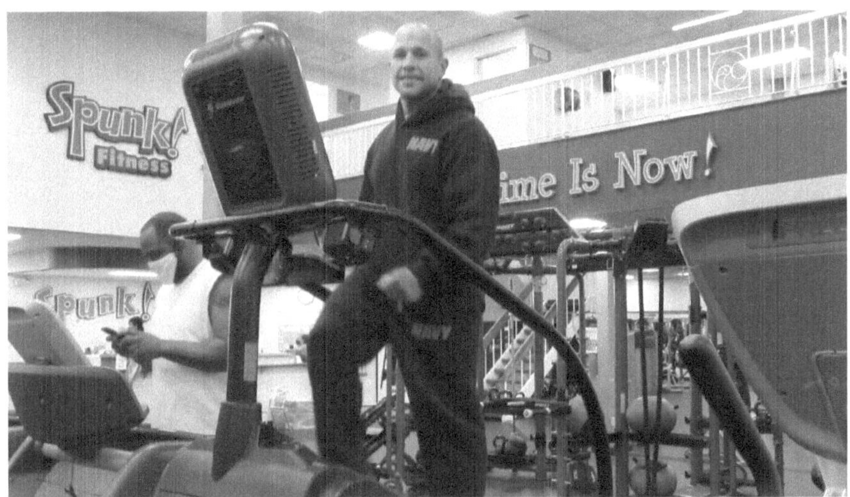

Climbing the stairs of a StairMaster

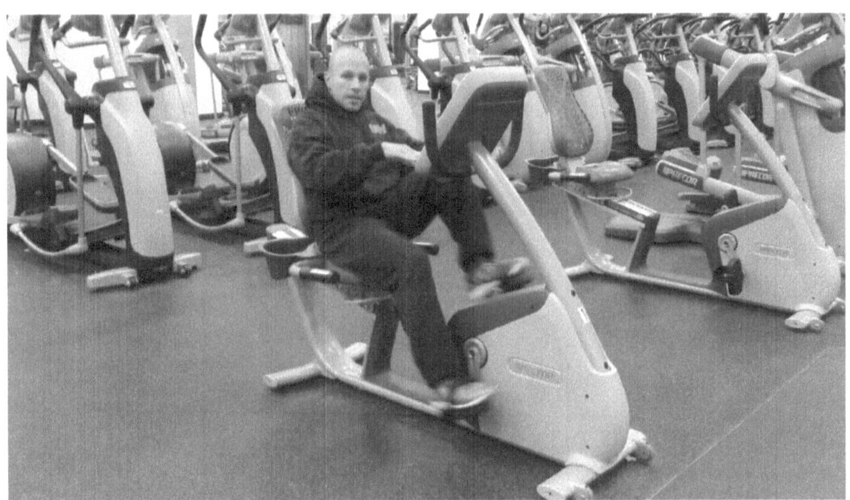

A stationary bike can be a valuable tool when it's cold outside.

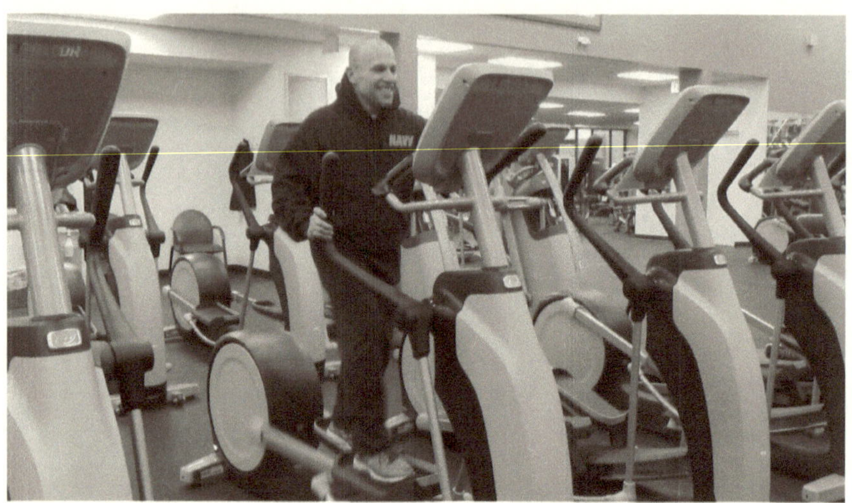

An elliptical can provide good aerobic movement for the arms.

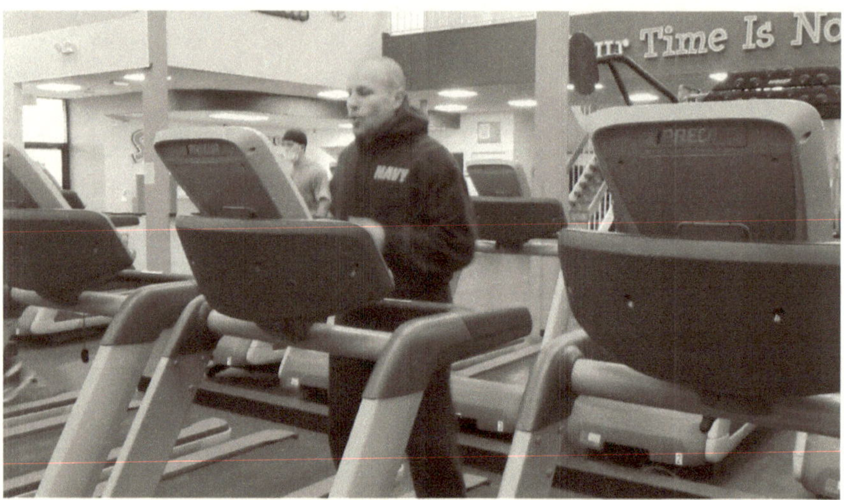

Take a break from the cold with a run on the treadmill.

Having variety provides more fun and additional growth to the aerobic or endurance training and exercise. A "steady state" approach can be a useful foundation for anyone who has been sedentary for a period of time or someone who is new to exercise. Only doing the same speed, intensity, and exercise for the months and years to come will not produce continued increases in fitness and health. With all the above options, alter intensity. Always remaining in the comfort zone will not continuously improve health and fitness. There are many who stick to the same "steady state" routine for years. Their body composition and fitness levels never improve despite their consistent exercise. The human body is highly intelligent. It adapts very quickly to the stress placed upon it. If there is not a new stimulus for the body to adapt to further physical or cardiovascular stress, improvements simply will not occur.

With any indoor exercise machine, there are a variety of manipulations that can be made to change intensity. Do not be lazy. Use the buttons to change speed and incline. One of the best ways to do this is through interval training. Below is a possible interval scenario for the treadmill:

<u>Speed</u> <u>Incline</u>

2 minutes 4.0 mph 2 percent
1 minute 6.0 mph 4 percent
2 minutes 5.0 mph 2 percent
1 minute 7.0 mph 4 percent
2 minutes 5.0 mph 2 percent
1 minute 7.5 mph 2 percent
2 minutes 4.5 mph 2 percent
1 minute 8.0 mph 2 percent
2 minutes 4.0 mph 4 percent
1 minute 8.5 mph 0 percent
2 minutes 4.0 mph 2 percent
5 minutes (easy pace for a cooldown with no incline)

Note: the workout above is not very long. It could easily be shorter or longer depending on the exercise capacity of the individual. Always remember that intensity and effort are more important than duration.

The example above is for a treadmill. A stationary bike can be monitored with speed and a measurement of resistance. Ellipticals measure speed and various levels of incline too. The StairMaster apparatus provides options to enhance speed, so it forces someone to climb the steps in a hurry. Whatever modality is being used, a creative approach should be used. Realize though that interval training is more advanced. Start with a specific plan and stick with it for one workout. Take note of how the body responded. In the next workout, raise intensity or cut back a little if needed. If rest or lack of sleep is an issue, modify the workout accordingly. Nothing is written in stone. Listen to the body and modify or adjust accordingly.

<u>An outdoor interval routine at the track could be the following examples</u>:

* Run straightaway at 50 percent to 75 percent speed.
* Jog-turn.
* This is done until at least one full mile is completed.

Note: This can also be done by running the turns fast and jogging straightaway. If the left side is facing in toward the field, try doing the opposite direction next time if possible.

<u>Here is a second option:</u>

* Jog 300 meters.
* Run 100 meters at 90 percent speed (basically a sprint but not quite full speed).
* Continue this for 1 to 2 miles (four to eight laps).

<u>Here's option three:</u>

* Jog 200 meters.
* Run 200 meters at 50 percent to 75 percent speed.
* Continue this sequence for 1 to 2 miles (four to eight laps).

Note: The track interval workouts above are for three nonconsecutive days. Track athletes would most likely be doing five or six days a week with the intensity for each day being different.

Other Possibilities

Distance runs can be quite creative. They can be performed on cross-country routes with uneven terrain at various speeds and incline. A grass surface is more comfortable than a concrete surface. The uneven terrain, however, will be a greater challenge for stability, most specifically at the ankle joint. Usually on a cross-country route, there is hill work—both up and down. Both are challenging in different ways. Running uphill will require greater strength, while going down, body control and awareness are needed. When going downhill, the tendency is to run faster. An adjustment in stride will be needed. The trail can provide greater stimulation for the body. Give it a try, and do not do what you are comfortable with all the time. It is when we get uncomfortable that we create the greatest benefit for the heart in the long run—pun intended.

Running on pavement is fine for many, but sometimes the joints could use a change of surface. Whatever the surface though, be creative and alter speed at various segments and do not be afraid to run up hills. Other running workouts are listed below:

This is option four:

* A 5K run on a cross-country trail with variation in the terrain. Goals can be set to accomplish this in fifteen, twenty, twenty-five, or thirty minutes, depending on your ability. Also, one day could be at twenty minutes, and the next workout could be at thirty for restorative purposes. A third day could be something in the middle or a different approach or activity altogether.

Here's option 5:

* Run on any surface outside for forty-five to sixty minutes. (This could be a steady-state run, but gradually pick up speed in future workouts or change running location for new challenges and scenery.)
* Run on any surface for thirty to forty-five minutes. (See above for similar details.)
* Run any surface for fifteen to thirty minutes. (This should be a more intense pace than usual.)

Note: three separate days are described above. More could be added depending on goals and recovery.

Note: every workout does not have to be a hard effort. The body does better with variation. Think of this. The greatest athletes at any sport do not train their hardest in every workout. No one can set a record in every training session. If anyone would try, they would ultimately never peak for their best performance for a specific day or event. Rather, they would simply overtrain and perhaps get injured.

<u>Other Considerations</u>

Running workouts mentioned above can be modified in a plethora of ways for any individual. You can add to them in time, speed, and effort or detract from them in all the same ways. The individual should know his or her body best—present level of fitness and health, what their goals are, previous or current injuries, and how they want exercise and training to change their life for the better. Most machine apparatuses, like a treadmill or elliptical, have a built-in feature that coincides with a heart monitor strap. A heart rate monitor device does not have to be used with an indoor exercise machine. A run outside can certainly be monitored for heart rate. There are a variety of watches that are very suitable for this. These implements are helpful to dictate intensity. Enhancing intensity is how we improve. Getting the heart rate raised to certain levels will create a stronger heart muscle. Any of the running workouts listed in this chapter can utilize a watch that monitors heart rate. Knowing how hard the heart is working can help awareness. This awareness can help anyone realize if training intensity should decrease, stay the same, or be escalated. Each workout can also have a goal-specific intensity level for heart rate too. A possible scenario is to have one day where a heart rate goal is 180. Of course, this level cannot be maintained for an entire workout. Perhaps two or three times, this target heart rate can be reached. It can be complimented with lower-intensity workloads that are longer in duration, providing recovery. A separate day can have a goal as 150 for the target heart rate. Again, at some point during the workout, this number is reached. How long and how often it is maintained or reached depend upon the level of the athlete or participant. A third day may have only 130 as the goal, and a fourth strives back for 170. The Karvonen formula may be used to help you know which numbers to attain, but do not forget the Karvonen formula, like other formulas for targeting heart rate, is not perfect. They may be as many as twenty beats off or even more. Studies from Hakki, Pollack, Leger, Blair, and Kaminsky all suggest 220-age is not the most ideal approach to begin to predict max heart rate and target heart rate zones.

<u>Not as Simple as the Numbers Say</u>

I heard someone question why watches and gadgets are even necessary tools when all we really have to do is just pay attention to how the body feels and responds. This is a logical question, and it does bring us to other interesting points. An advanced athlete or fitness enthusiast has a great sense of bodily awareness. They can dictate, alter, and modify intensity very easily as is appropriate for the training session and specific goals. A heart rate monitor may say one thing, but they adjust to the innate wisdom of the body rather than a heart rate monitor. Another consideration is the "linear logic" of exercise physiology—run faster to increase heart rate and run slower to decrease heart rate. Is this how things always materialize? Examples exist where the trajectory of the heart is not always a straight line. The heart sometimes beats too fast for the current pace or activity. Sending oxygen to the working muscles is not the only job of the heart. The heart also manages body temperature. Heart rate climbs, but it may not be because of how hard the leg muscles are working—at least not entirely. A third item is the loss of bodily fluid. The heart beats faster as perspiration increases. This is in concert with blood volume decreasing—the heart goes faster to adjust for this. As this is occurring, a monitor may indicate that we are working harder, but we are not necessarily working harder in the leg muscles. This could make someone think they should go slower because they are in sync with their monitor, but they may not be paying attention to how they actually feel. Experience, body awareness, and an honest assessment on how one feels are important attributes to exercise too. Heart rate monitors can be a helpful tool, but we shouldn't be a slave to them—especially when working toward maintaining target heart rate zones.

Many think of their heart rate monitor as a tool for observing how hard the heart is working. The goal can be getting the heart rate up to maximum levels or near there. When the heart is working harder, it gets stronger, right? Yes, this is correct, but there is something else to be aware of. No matter the person, there is a maximum heart rate specific to the individual. Dr. Fritz Hagerman, who studied world-class rowers for three decades, observed elite athletes with a max heart rate of 220 and others with a max heart rate of 160. Maximum heart rate does not have to do with a lot of items, including our conditioning level. There is an important genetic component to realize. The size of the heart varies from person to person. Generally, a smaller heart beats more often compared to a larger one, which beats more slowly as it ejects more blood with each beat.

Accuracy cannot be overemphasized. I recall many people at fitness facilities telling me the exercise machine they were using, through my twenty plus years in the industry now, gives them a very high heart rate reading, but they feel great, and the intensity is easy. I told them what I will tell you right now—trust your body before you trust any machine. There are many gadgets out there and more formulas than are needed. They can be helpful, but they are all secondary to the innate wisdom of the human body. They will not deliver 100 percent accuracy. A true max heart rate can be determined by a stress test. Two examples are the Balke and Bruce treadmill stress tests. These are important for another reason too. Stress tests do not necessarily determine coronary artery disease according to Aristotelis Vlahos M.D. More accurately, a stress test considers blood flow to the heart and determines if it is sufficient. In this example, an echocardiogram is monitoring the heart, and trained personnel are on standby to decipher what is going on.

Frank-Starling Mechanism

Ernest Frank and Otto Starling were two exercise physiologists who made an interesting contribution in understanding max heart rate. Max heart rate is not attained simply with a 400-meter sprint or an all-out running effort up a hill. The first response of the heart to an intense challenge is to add stroke volume and not stroke frequency. Stroke volume is a measure of blood the heart pumps with each beat. Frank and Starling noted in their study of the heart that when the volume of blood increases in the ventricles, so does the length of the cardiac muscle fibers. This creates a situation where the muscle fibers of the heart work in greater unison—forcing more blood to be ejected with every beat. A slower heart rate is the result. This regulation of the heart is conducted by the sinus node, which is a component of the nervous system that excites the heart to contract. Now if someone is using a heart rate monitor, they may be surprised that the heart rate does not indicate a higher number because the effort exerted seems to indicate that. Something else does increase—cardiac output. This is stroke volume times stroke frequency. Therefore, oxygenated blood is going to the working muscles in a greater amount. If using a heart rate monitor, something interesting is revealed. The heart rate appears lower than expected while the effort being exerted is causing heavy breathing and perhaps some initial fatigue.

Further Explanation

The experience described above does not last. This segment is different for everyone. The training level and ability of the participant will dictate the cardiorespiratory system getting the optimum oxygen to where it is needed. As always, with any physical activity, a greater demand for oxygen will be met with greater heart rate. This is inevitable. Before the elevation of heart rate though, there is a period where muscles tighten up due to a rapid buildup of lactic acid. This is due to working muscles being emptied of oxygen. At some point, the cardiorespiratory system will acclimate to the challenge, and it will be smooth sailing for you. Then an ideal situation for using a heart rate monitor occurs because the heart rate, goals, and/or target heart rate zone chosen for that workout, and effort exerted should all coincide. This then reverts back to the linear logic of exercise physiology because the monitor and effort reveal what is expected.

Another Interesting Note

Each bodily system may respond differently depending on the workout. This is referring to the lungs (respiratory), heart (cardiovascular), and skeletal muscle tissue doing most of the work for an exercise. One example to consider is a long run at a moderate pace. The following day's workout demonstrates tired muscles in the legs. The heart and lungs are not fatigued from the previous aerobic workout. A monitor reveals that the heart is not working that hard, but the skeletal muscles feel very differently because of the long run the day before. The leg muscles may not be able to work much harder to get heart rate up. This is a reminder that it is important to trust the body and not be overly concerned that a specific heart rate range must be attained.

Staying Mindful

There are a plethora of movements and activities that are good for the development of the heart. The ideas and points stressed above are for more than running. Walking, hiking, biking, triathlon, skating, swimming, group exercise classes, and rowing are all possibilities to train the heart muscle with monitors or by simple body awareness and other strategies. Remember, change things up with exercise selection and intensity. The body does well with variety and changes in intensity. Even an elite Olympic middle distance runner will benefit from easy workouts for restoration and additional speed and strength work on occasion. In the next section, we will consider strengthening the heart with other creative possibilities.

Circuit Training Options

A number of years ago, there was a writer from *Strength and Health* magazine named John McCallum. He popularized a circuit training approach called peripheral heart action (PHA). The concept considered a series of exercises that were very different in their emphasis. A group of exercises may have exercises that overlap, but with PHA training, the next exercise is unrelated to the previous. Circulation is enhanced throughout the entirety of the body and not just one area. Other attributes of PHA included enhancing the strength of the heart and lungs while also improving muscular definition. It is believed the idea for PHA originally came from bodybuilders Bob Gajda and Sergio Oliva of the 1960s. Below is an example of a PHA routine:

1) Ball leg curl × 20
2) Dumbbell bench press × 10
3) Barbell squat × 10
4) Barbell bent-over row × 10
5) Body weight calf raise × 20
6) Dumbbell side deltoid raise × 10

A one- to two-minute rest can follow the completion of this group of exercises. It can be repeated for three to six rounds. Take note of the diversity of the exercises that follow each other. Remember, if you do two sets consecutively of the same movement, you are not doing peripheral heart action training. Also, after one exercise is completed, go immediately to the next.

Below are picture demonstrations for each of the exercises listed above.

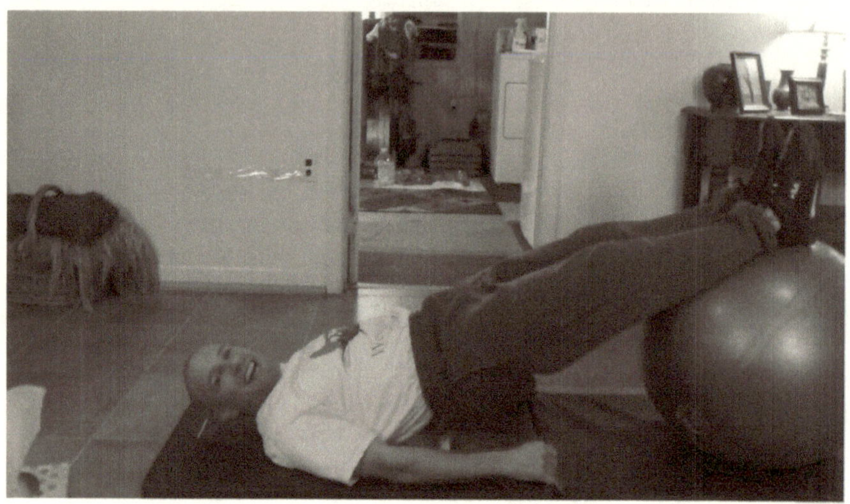

The start of the ball leg curl

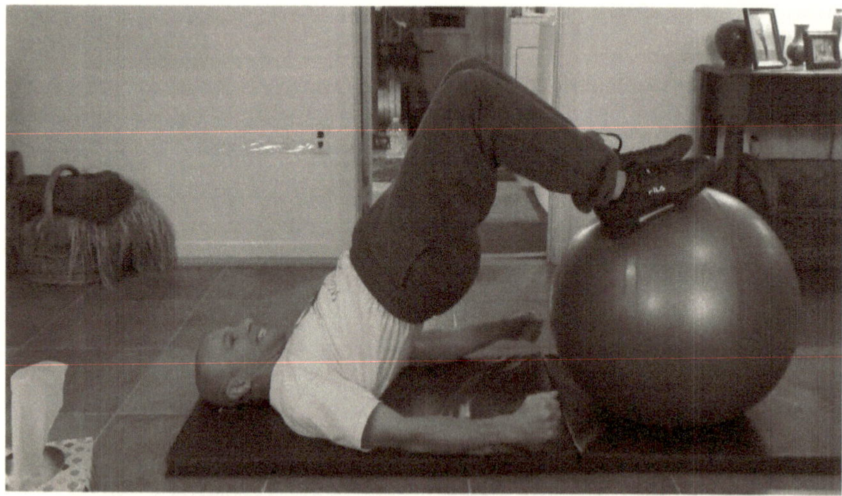

The top of the ball leg curl. From this position, the legs extend back out to where they started, and the reps continue until completed.

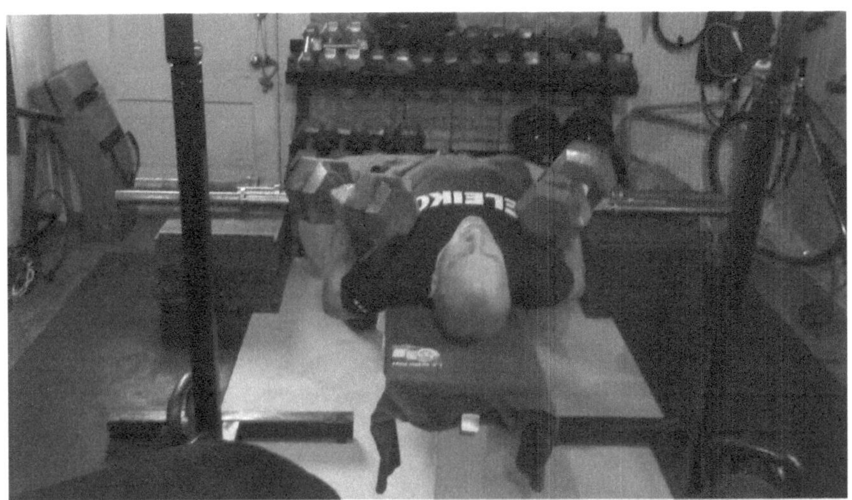

This is the starting position for the dumbbell bench press.

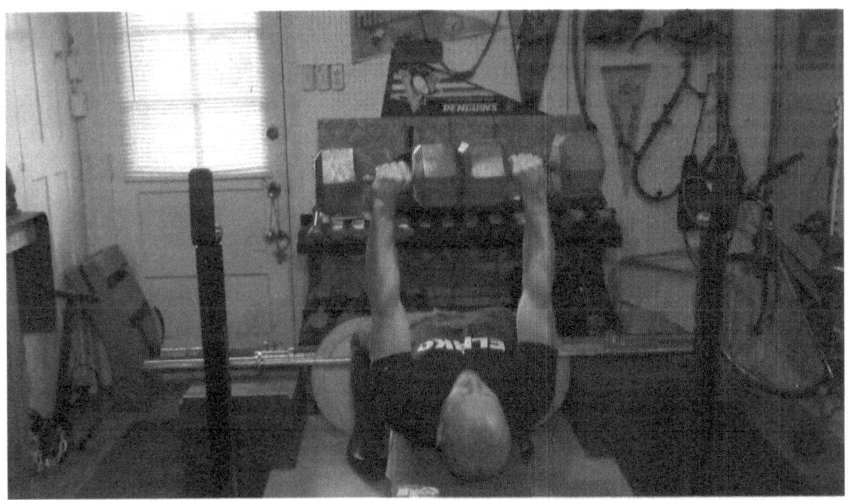

The top position for the dumbbell bench press. Come
back down for a full range of motion.

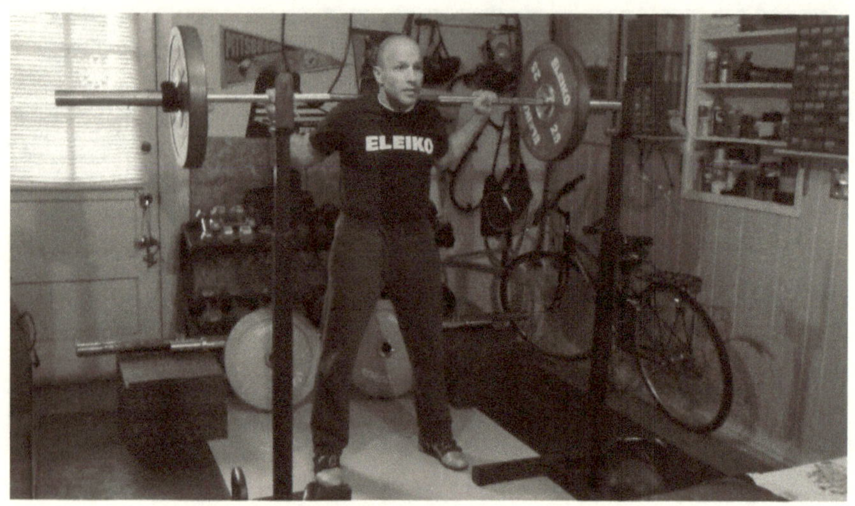

Starting position for barbell squat

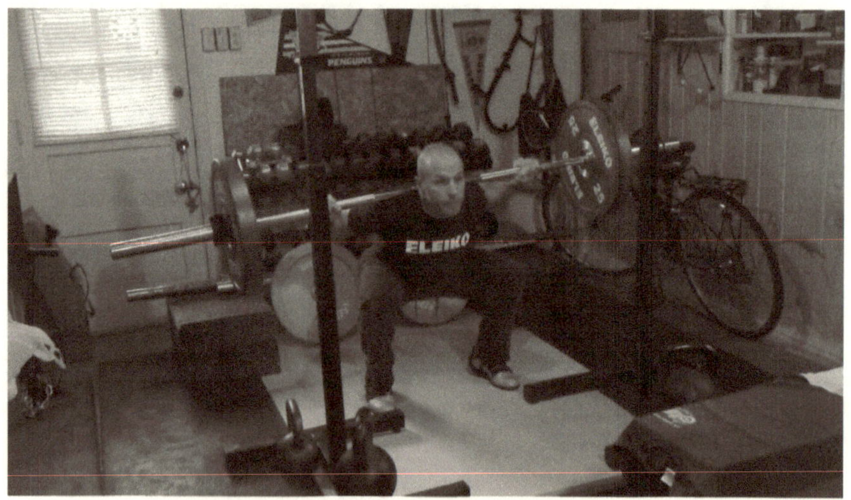

The bottom position for barbell squat. Notice the
feet flared for a comfortable stance.

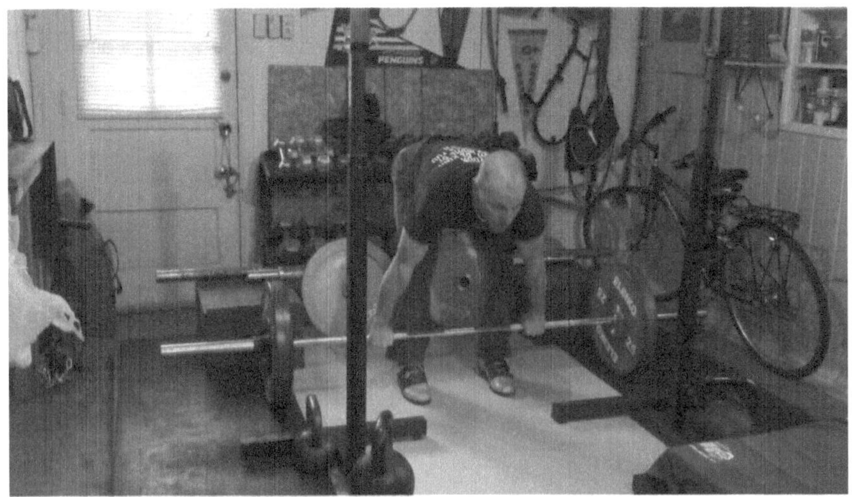

This is the start for the barbell bent-over row. Notice the straight back position with eyes slightly up.

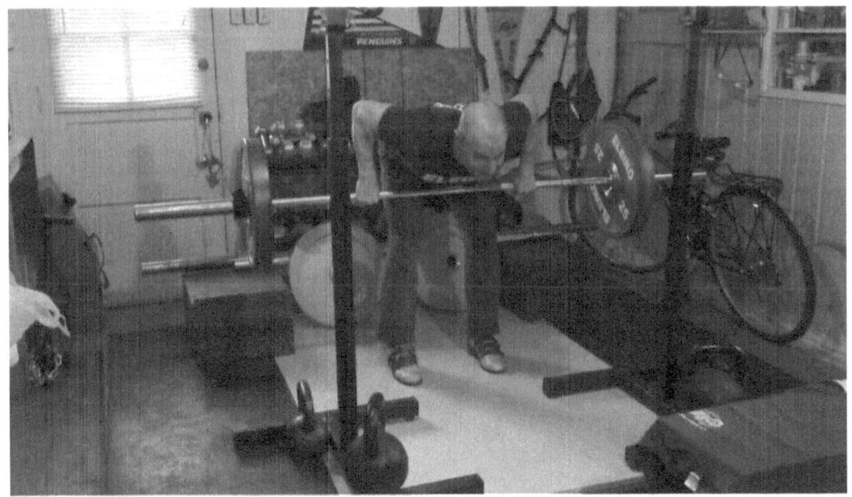

Completing the rowing action. The knees in this exercise are slightly bent as the back remains straight.

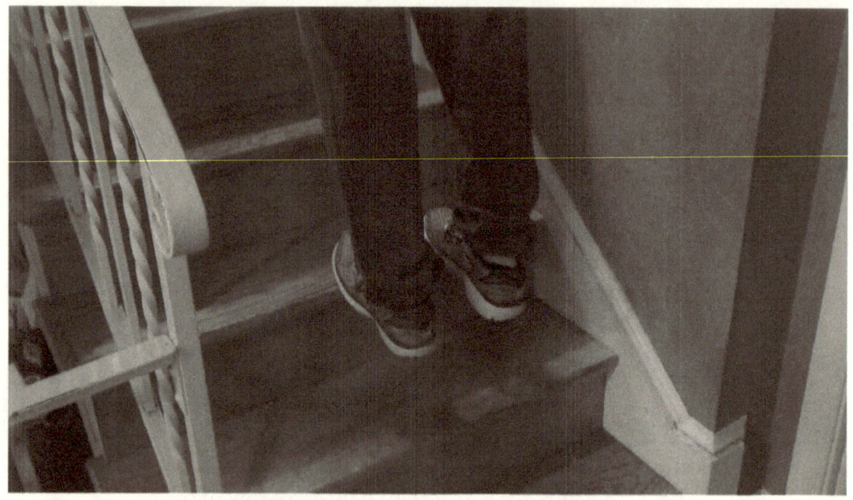

Prestretch position to start calf raise.

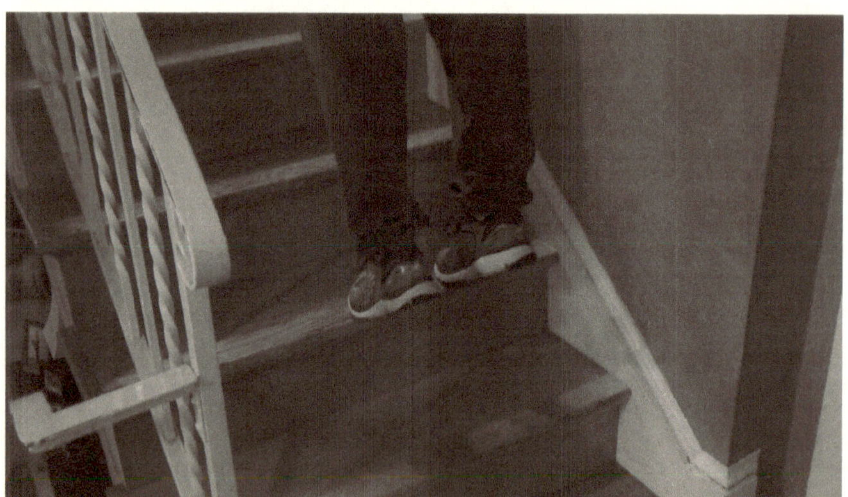

Perform the calf raise with as much range of motion
as possible at the start and top position.

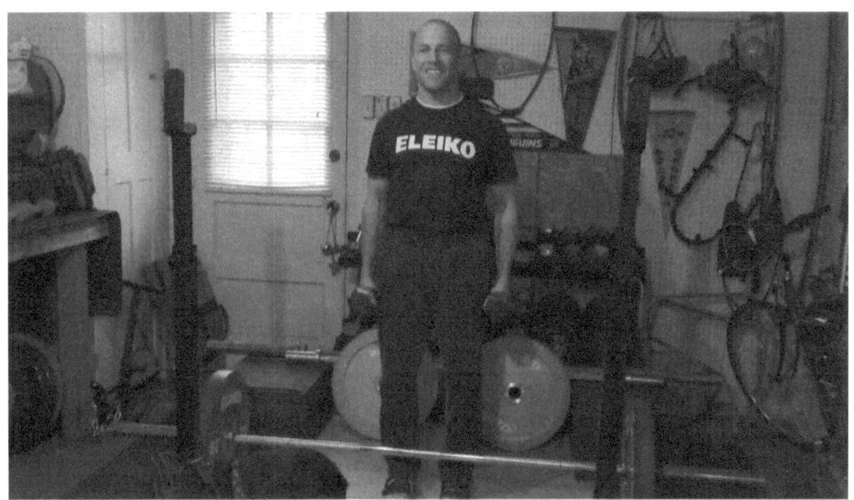

Side delt raise starting position

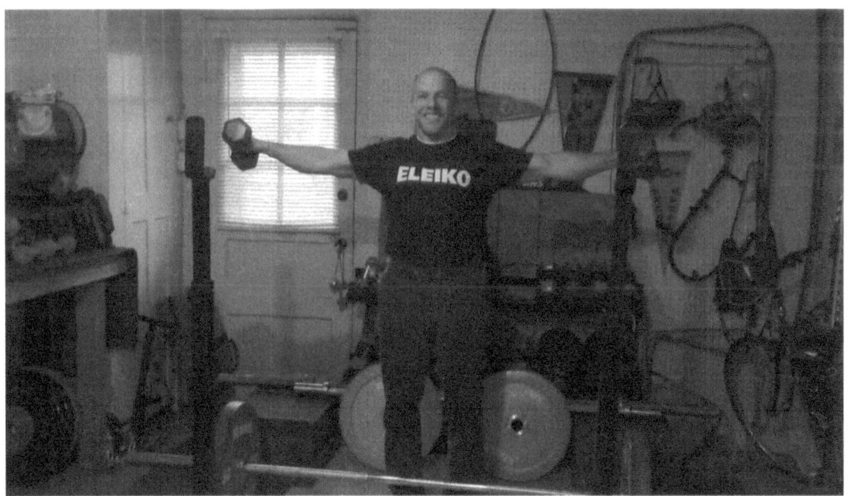

Get the dumbbells to shoulder height.

The next group covers a traditional circuit. Circuit training is considered a conditioning program. It may consist of only weight training, but it is not limited to weight training. Consecutive exercises may overlap to the extent that the muscles being worked are in a similar body area or that blood flow is being increased to the same or similar area of the body for consecutive sets. The traditional circuit includes the following example:

1) Step-ups (alternating × 10 each leg; 20 total)
2) Dumbbell reverse fly × 10
3) Renegade row (alternating × 10 each arm; 20 total)
4) Donkey kicks × 20
5) Barbell curl × 10
6) Dips × 10
7) Pull-up × 8
8) One-leg Romanian dead lift × 10
9) Push jack × 20
10) Bench jumps × 20

Pictures for each of these are listed next.

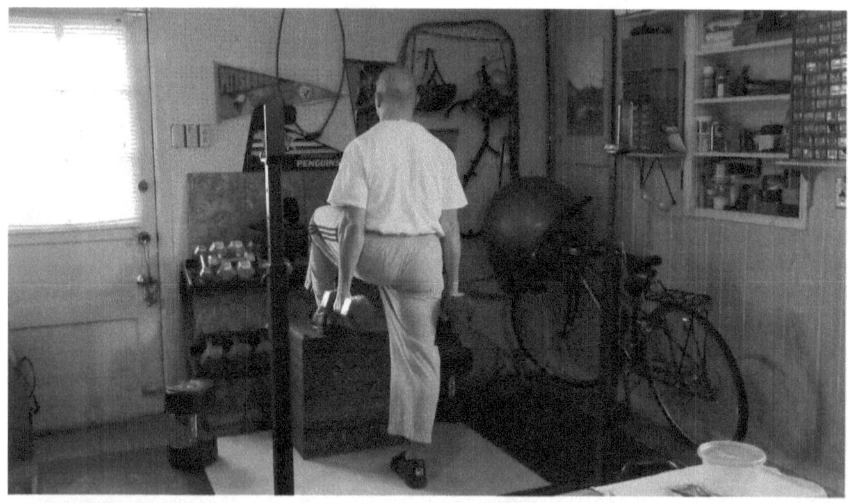

This is the step-up exercise being performed with a dumbbell in each hand.

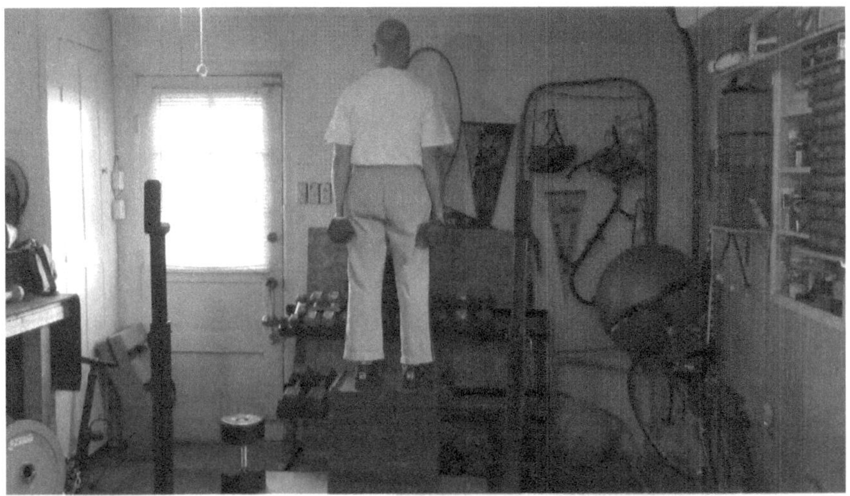

From here, you should step down with the same leg that stepped up first followed by the other leg and then have the other leg start for the next rep.

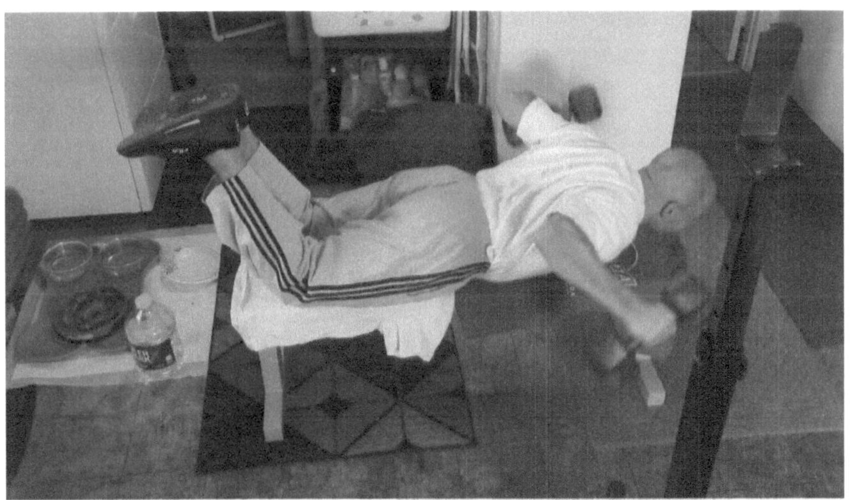

For the dumbbell reverse fly, start with dumbbells under bench and then perform a reverse fly. Notice the elbows are bent.

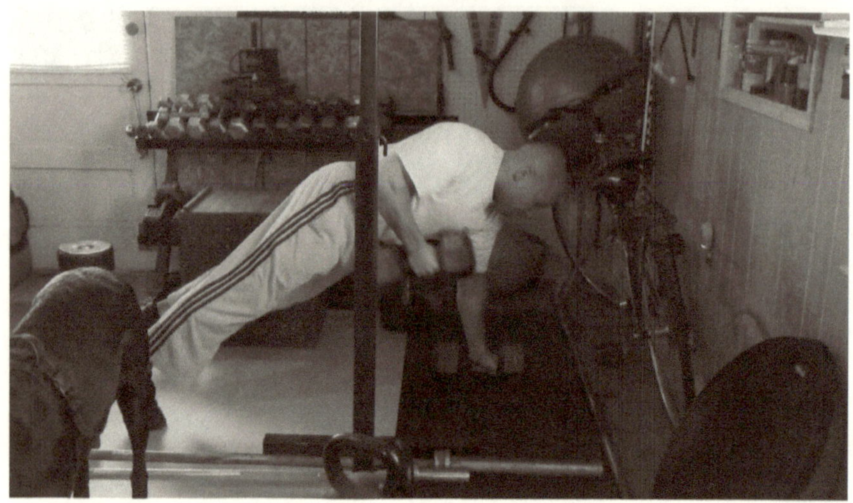

The renegade row is done from a plank position. The abdominal
wall stabilizes as a rowing action is performed on alternating sides.
Keep the elbow close to the side as the row is performed.

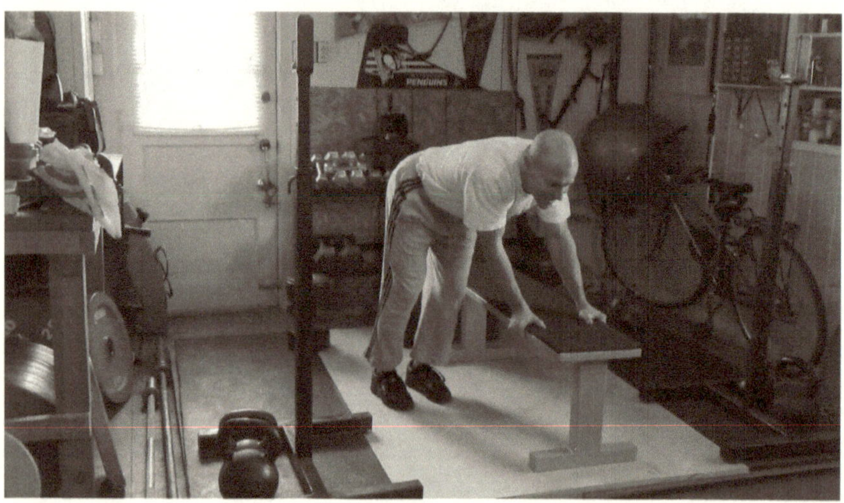

The donkey kicks begin on one side of the bench.

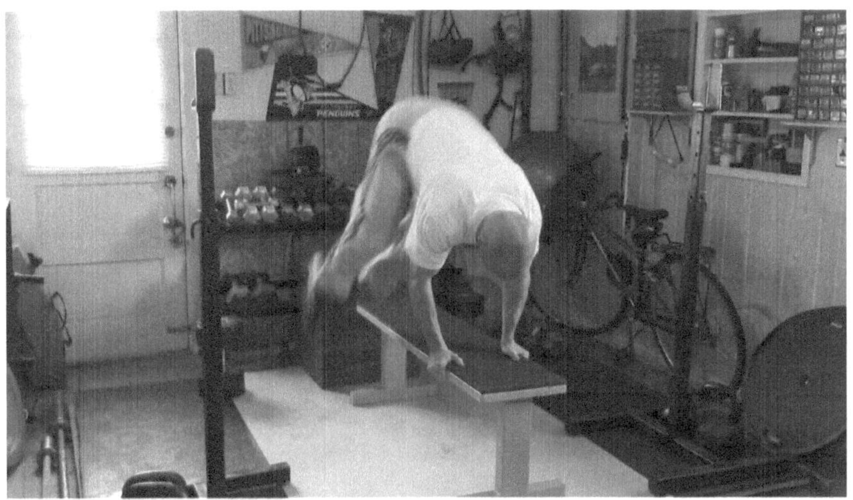

With stability through the shoulders, a powerful leaping
action is performed with the lower body.

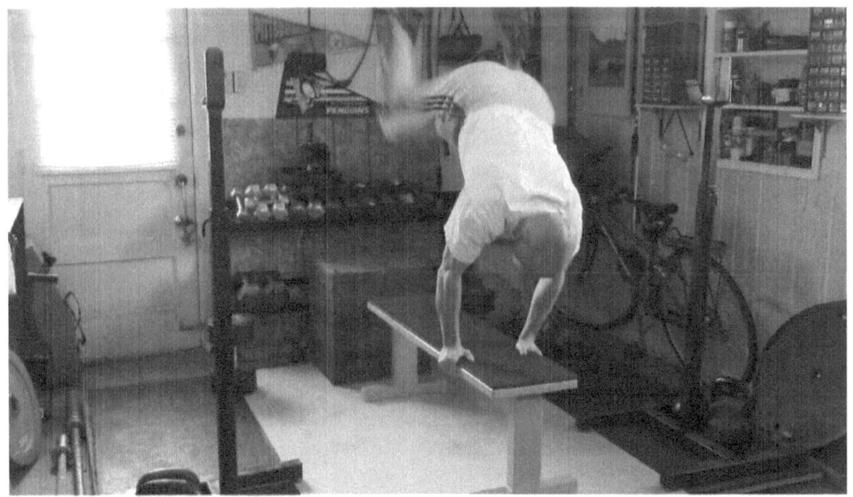

The legs are then kicked into the sky.

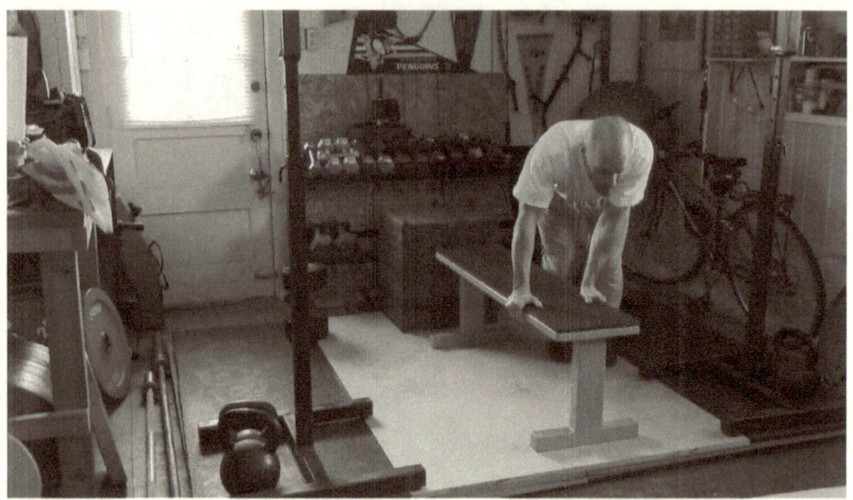

A safe landing happens on the opposite side, and the powerful pace continues until all reps are completed.

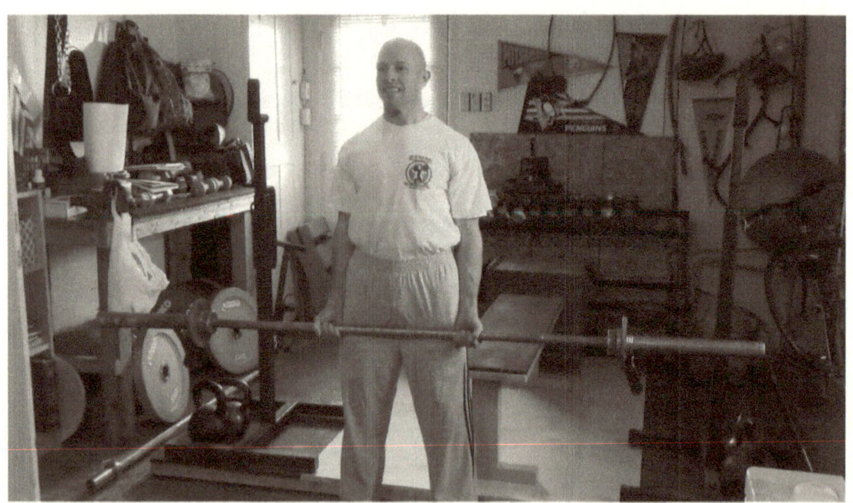

This depicts the start of the barbell curl.

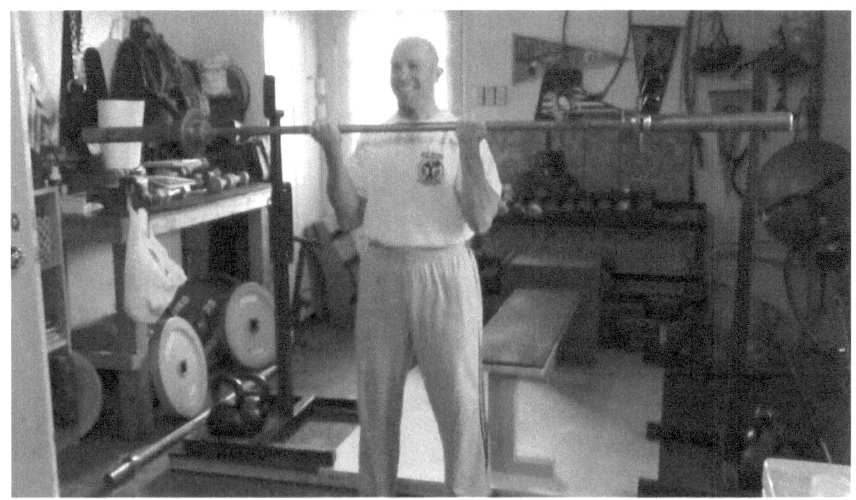

This is the barbell curl at the top position.

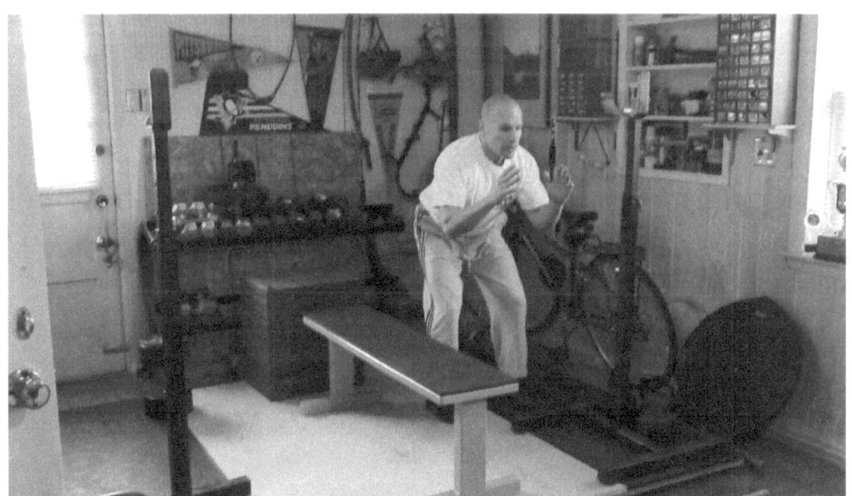

Bench jumps starting position

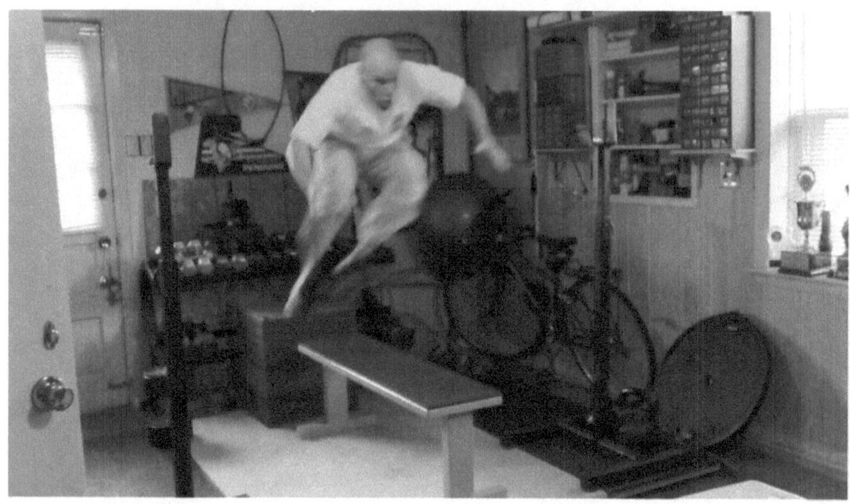

Bench jumps are an explosive movement. Once you land on the other side of the bench, explode back up to the opposite side immediately. This is continued until all reps are completed.

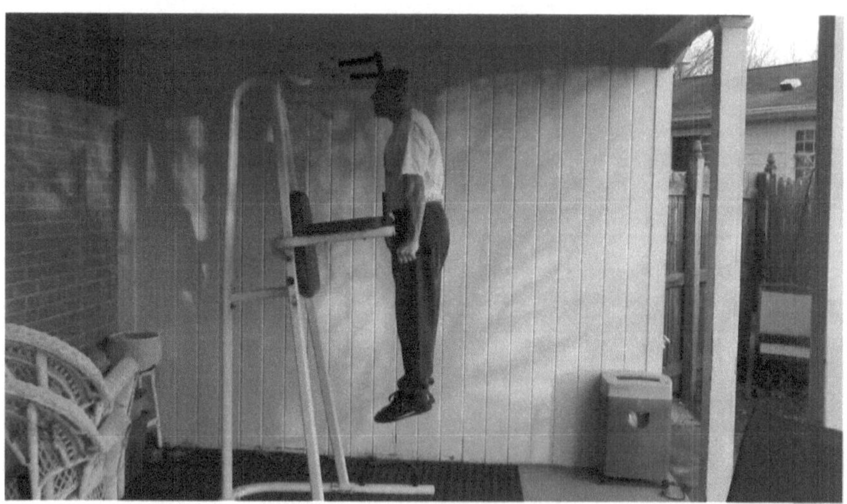

Dip exercise starting position

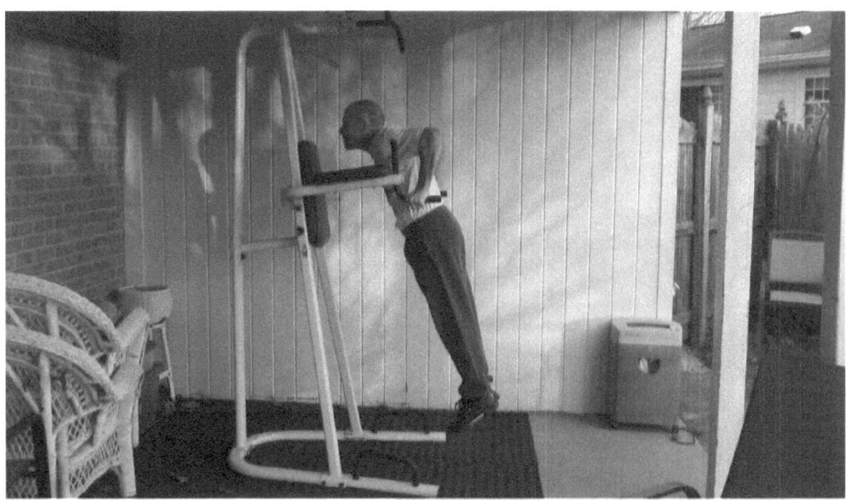

Try to get to ninety degrees at the elbows.

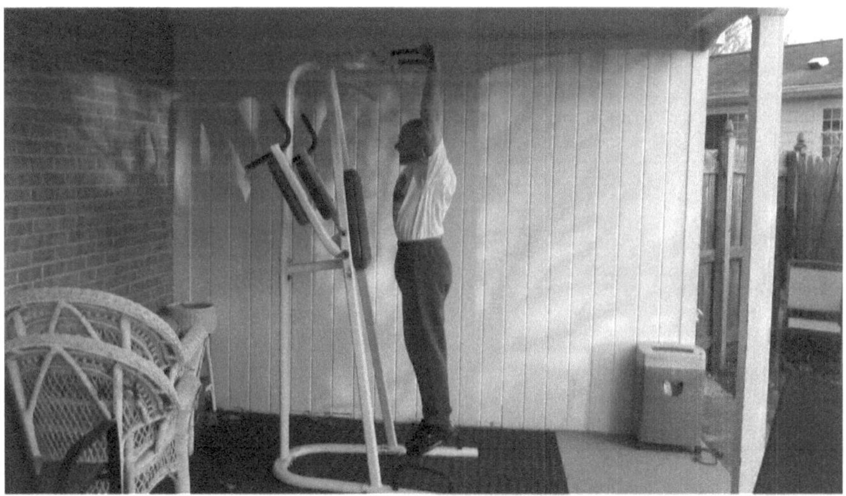

The pull-ups begin with a stretch through the latissimus dorsi
(large muscle of the back). This is a wonderful complimentary move
to the dips because of the opposing muscles being worked.

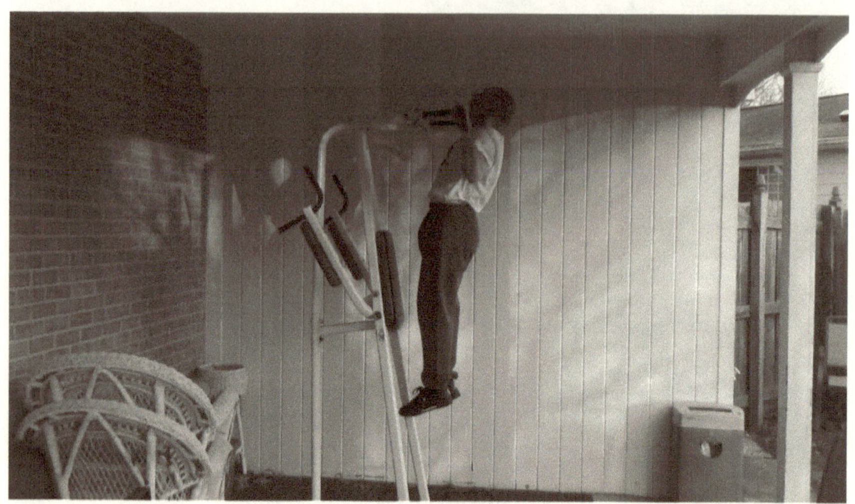

Pull-ups should finish with the chin being close to level
with the position of the hands or slightly above.

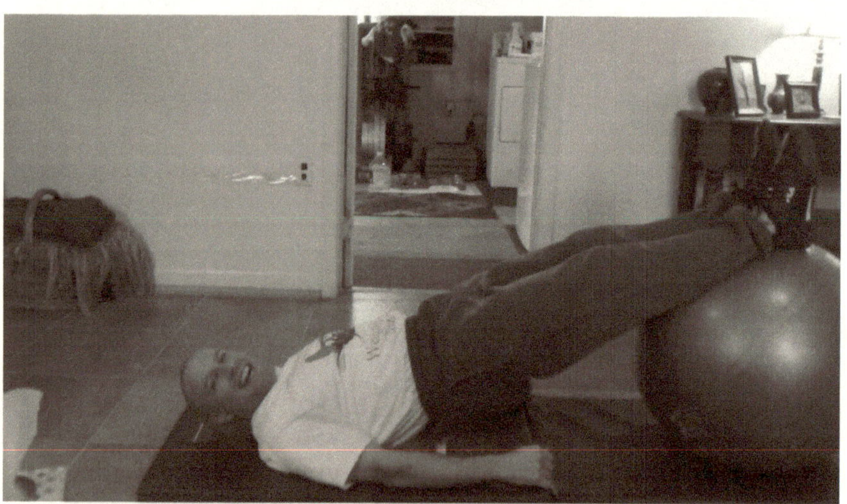

The ball leg curl begins with a hip extension.

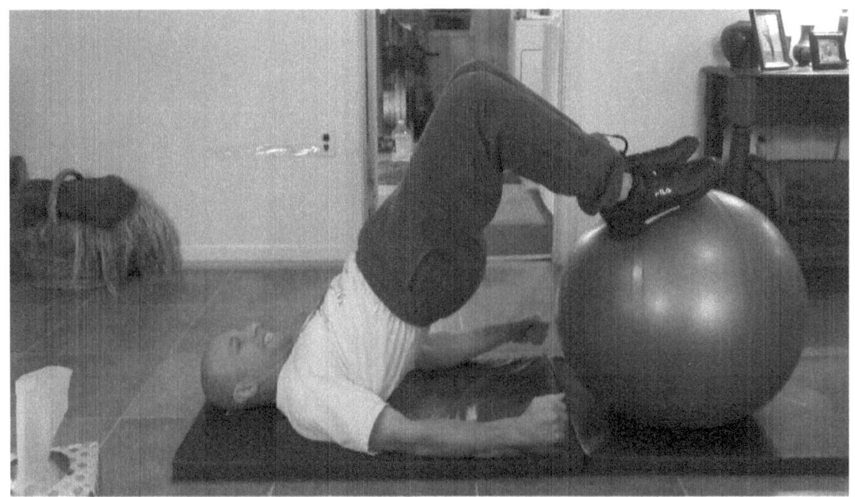

Notice the knee flexion at the top of this exercise.

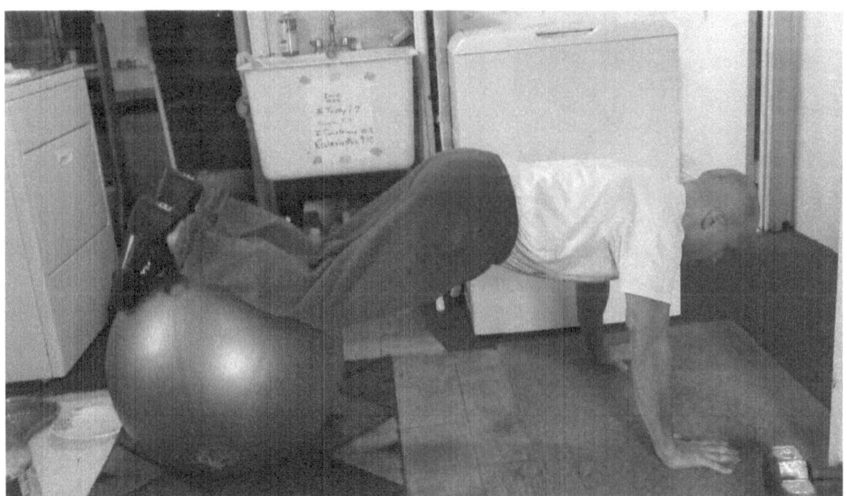

The start of the push jack

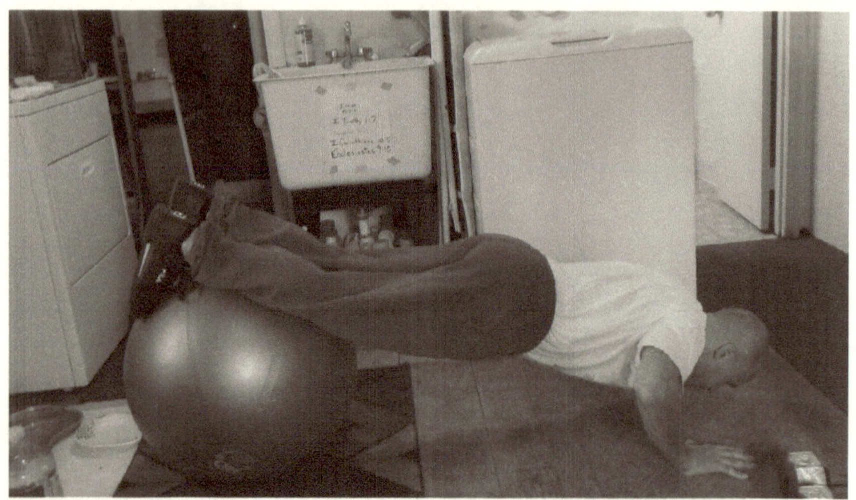

A push-up is performed in the middle portion of the exercise.

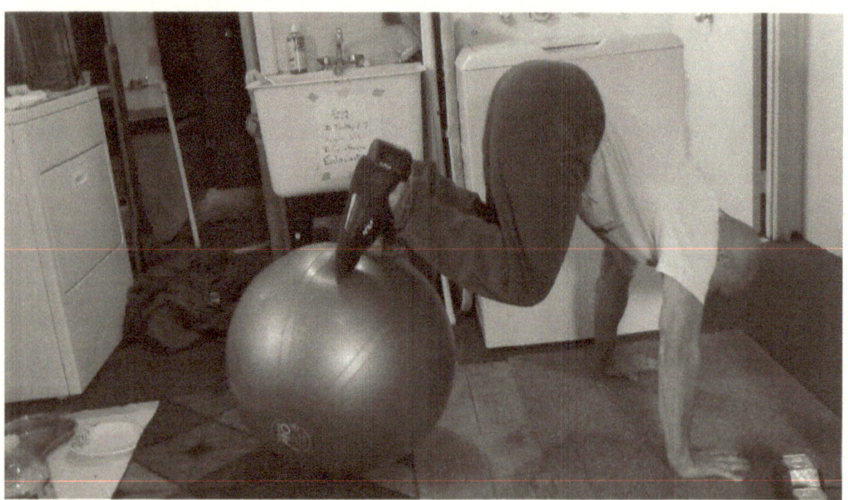

As you finish the push-up, bring the knees to the chest in
the top position and repeat until reps are completed.

Another option for circuit training can be accomplished with the same implement for each exercise. A kettlebell is a wonderful tool for this. The approach is simple, sweet, and highly time-efficient. You have one kettlebell and maybe another on standby if you feel a weight change is needed. You have a circuit of five exercises all at the same station with nowhere to run and hide. There is no rest in between, but you should rest for at least two minutes at the completion of the five kettlebell exercises. As many as five rounds can be completed for this circuit. Keep in mind with a circuit like this, there is a lot of overlap because each exercise can be considered a total body exercise. This is sometimes referred to as intermuscular coordination—the muscular system working as a team. One possible kettlebell circuit is listed below:

1) Swing × 10
2) Get up × 5
3) Power clean × 10
4) Power jerk × 10
5) Diagnol × 10

Pictures for each of these are listed below:

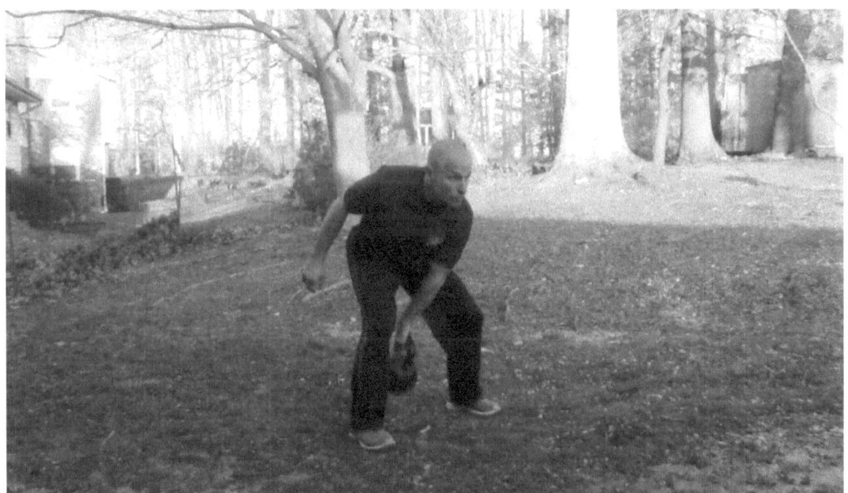

The swing begins with a swinging action between the knees. I like to orient my elbow outward at the start of the movement. This is a helpful technique that enhances advanced kettlebell exercises, but it is not necessary.

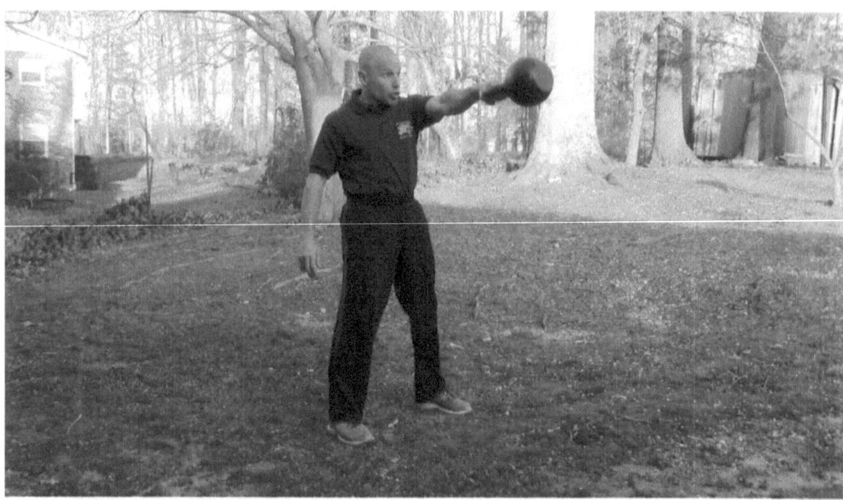

A powerful hip extension occurs, and the body finishes tall
with the arm extended out to chin height. The kettlebell never
touches the ground until all reps are completed. Each arm is done
individually, but a two-hand swing is a modification if needed.

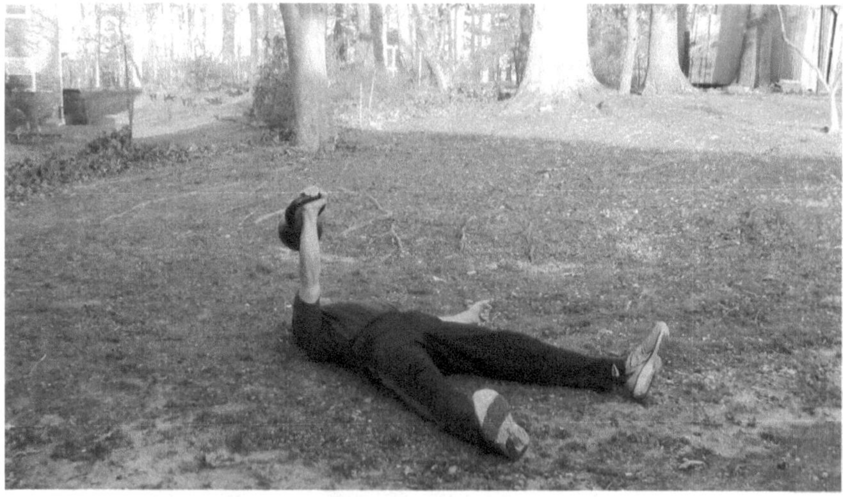

The get-up exercise begins as shown above. The eyes
should never lose focus on the kettlebell.

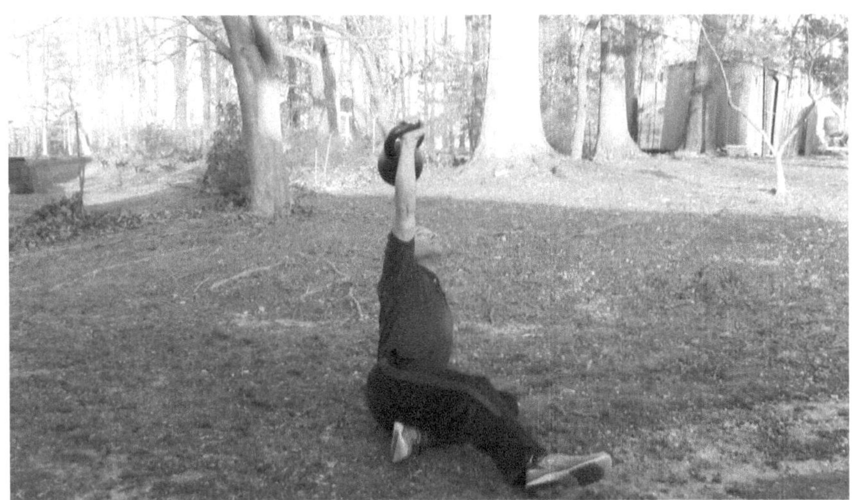

Notice the progression of the get-up as the right leg gets out in front of the body and left leg goes underneath the hips. Take note of the shoulder, elbow, and wrist all lining up with eyes focused on the bell. The left hand is starting to aid the movement by pushing into the ground.

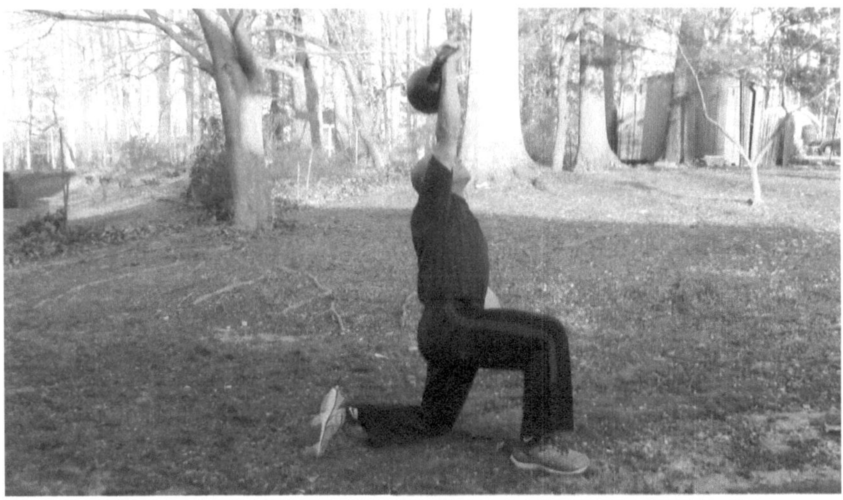

The get-up progression continues here into a split squat position with the right arm extended and right leg out in front. Notice again that the shoulder-to-wrist structure has not been broken.

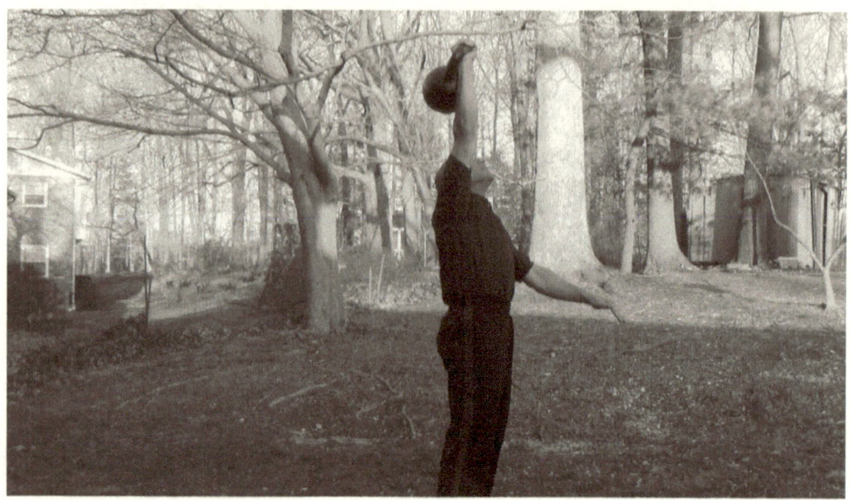

Here, the whole body straightens out, and feet come together. This completes the portion of the exercise coming off the ground.

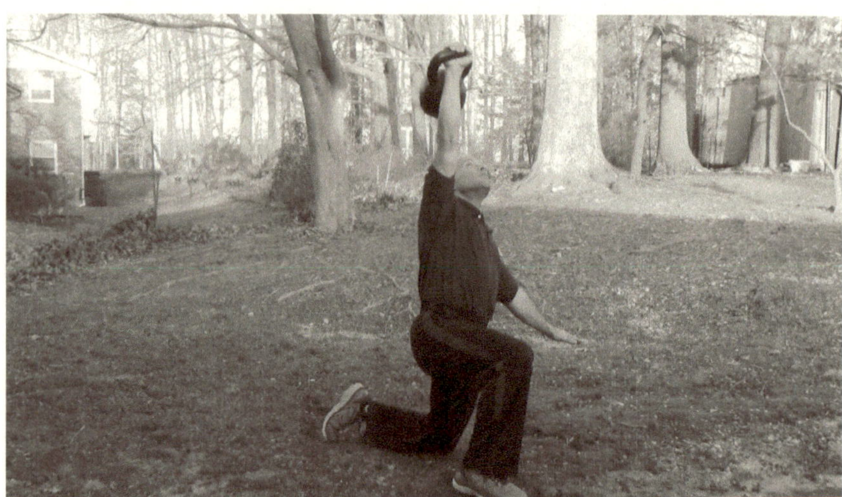

The body then lowers back to the ground under control. Notice the left hand getting ready to brace the body back to the ground. Each repetition finishes exactly how it started—lying back down with kettlebell extended over chest. The exercise is repeated on the other side in the opposite format.

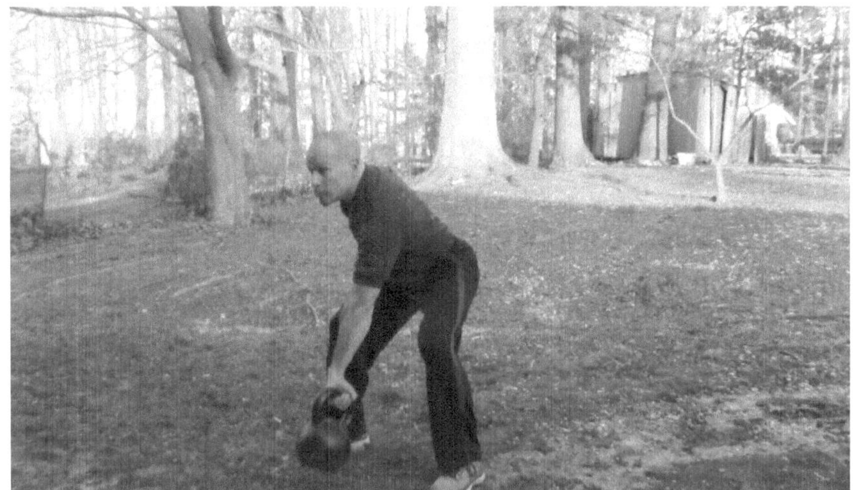

Here, we have the beginning of the power clean. It begins like the swing.
However, the kettlebell does not swing away from the body. It is pulled
up close after the initial swing between the knees. Notice again the
orientation of the elbow outward in the photo above. This helps ensure
the weight remains close to the body during the power clean movement.

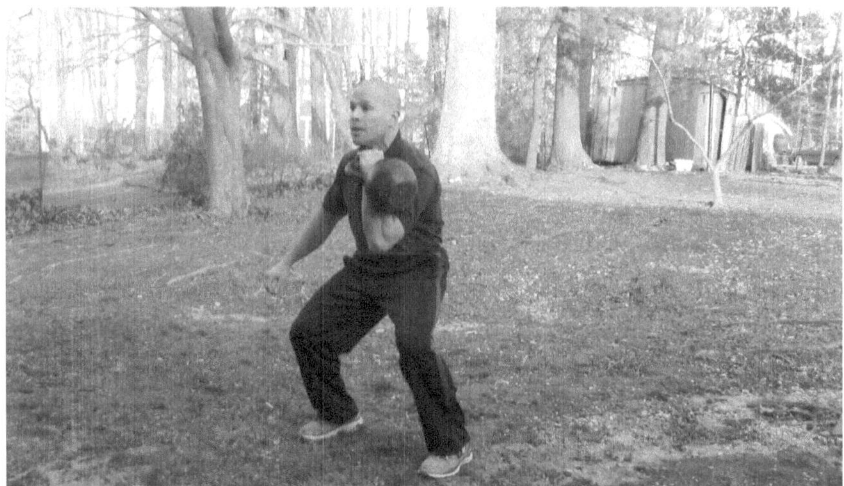

The power clean has weight finishing in the rack position as shown above. Be
mindful that the elbow to wrist create a straight line in this position. From
here, stand tall and repeat all reps without having the weight touch the ground.

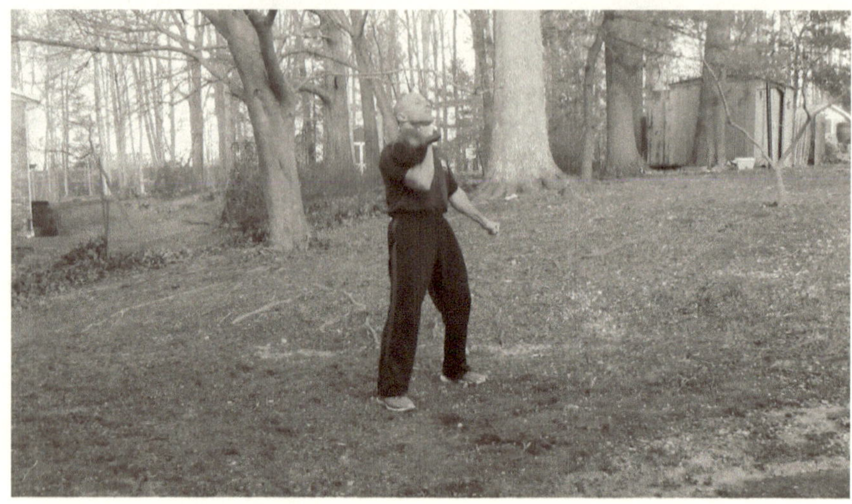

The power jerk begins standing tall in the rack position.
Notice that this is where the power clean finishes.

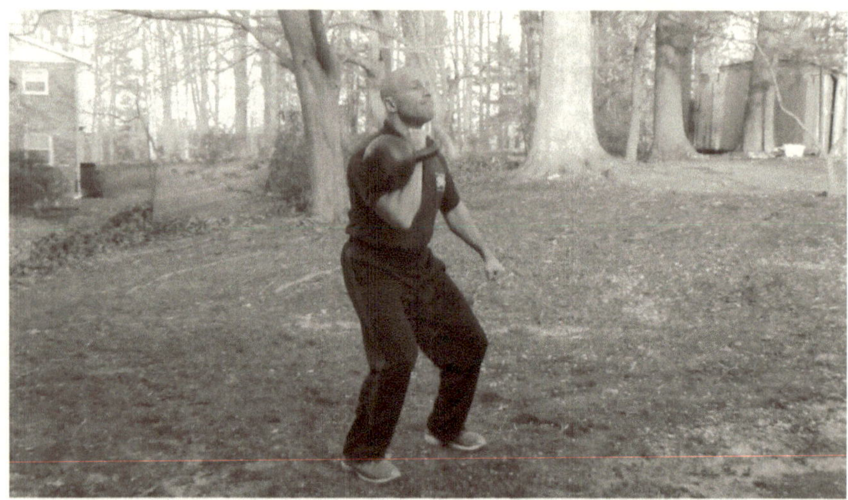

For the power jerk, the knees begin to bend. From here, there is
a powerful explosive movement upward as shown below.

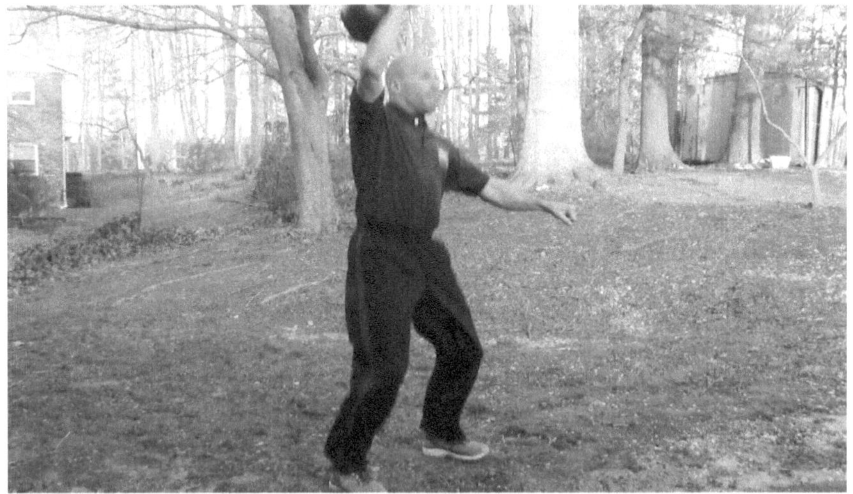

The body extends as the legs drive the kettlebell up.

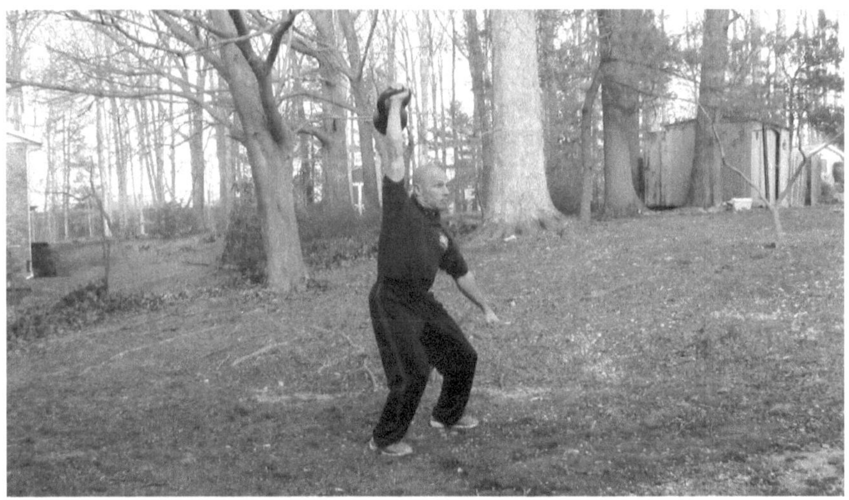

As the kettlebell finishes in full extension overhead, the hips
and knees dip back under the weight. Then they straighten out
again with weight remaining in full extension overhead.

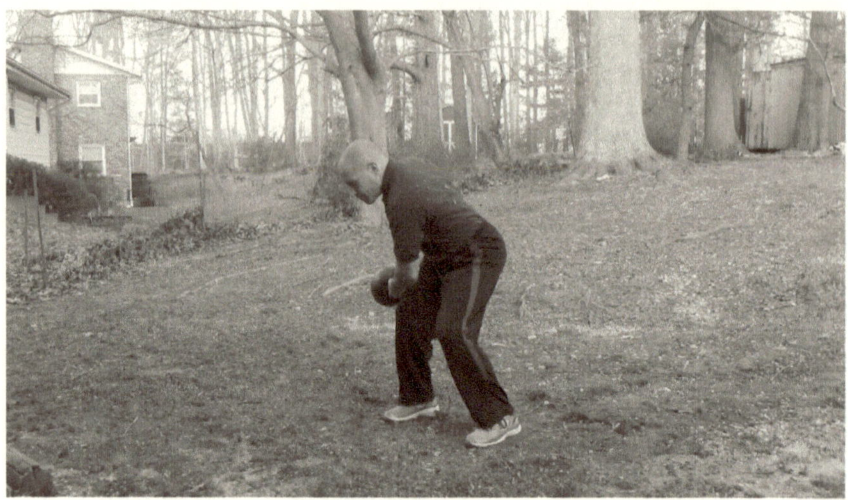

The kettlebell diagnol starts with the weight outside one knee.

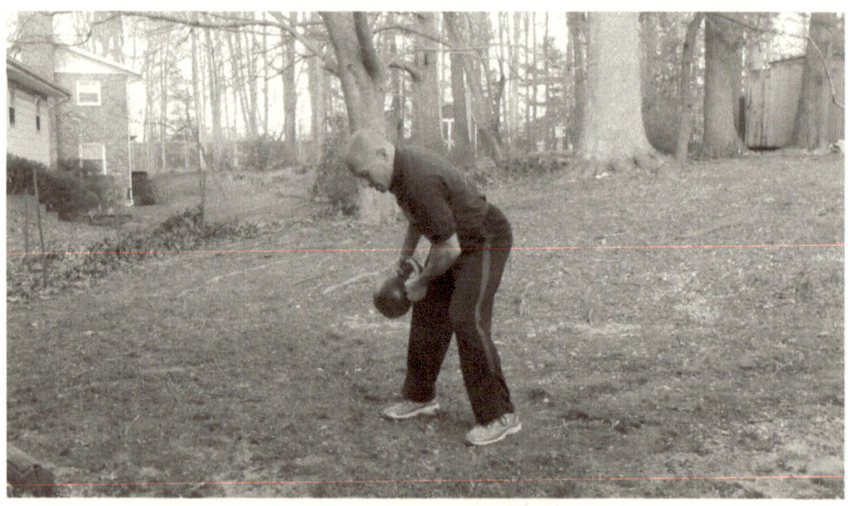

It progresses across the body. This movement
activates the abdominal wall and hips.

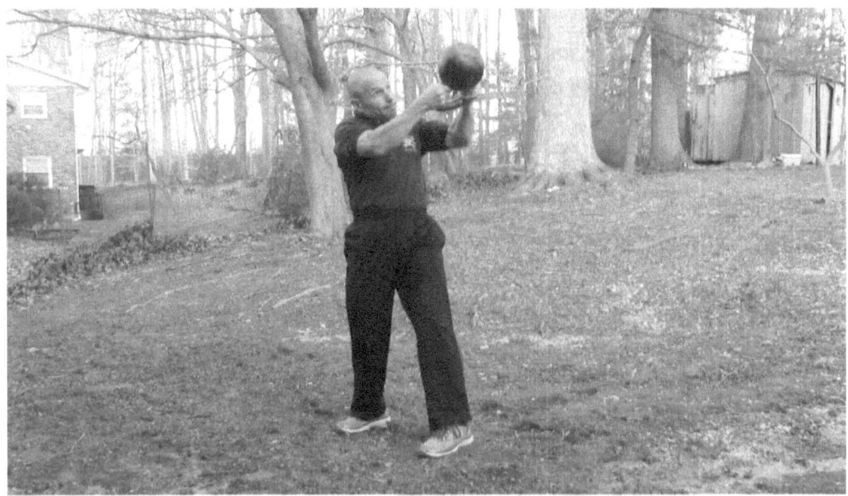

It finishes accelerating the kettlebell to the upper opposite corner of the body.

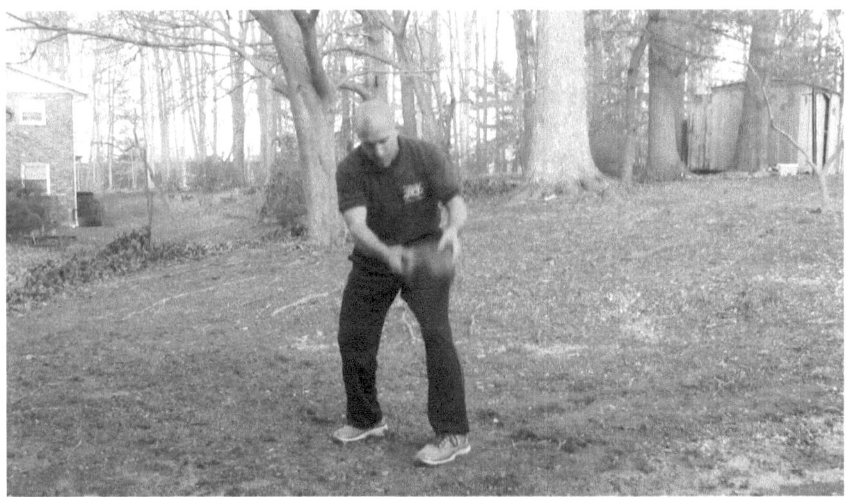

The kettlebell then returns to original position under control. It accelerates, going upward across the body, and then decelerates, going back outside the knee where the exercise was initiated.

With circuit training, variety and creativity have no limits. Dr. Al Sears, director of the Center for Health and Wellness in South Florida, has developed an approach he refers to as PACE (Progressively Accelerating Cardiopulmonary Exertion). This approach is done primarily with body weight exercises, but it can also be done with different machines too like an elliptical or rower. PACE utilizes intervals. There are short segments of high intensity followed by lower intensity levels for recovery. As always, the level of intensity is different for everyone. One example of a PACE routine is described below:

2 minutes: march or jog in place
30 seconds: regular jumping jacks
1 minute: march or jog in place
30 seconds: jumping jacks in sagittal plane
1 minute: march or jog in place
30 seconds: jumping jacks in transverse plane
1 minute: march or jog in place
30 seconds: burpees
1 minute: march or jog in place
30 seconds: mountain climbers
1 minute: march or jog in place
30 seconds: squats
1 minute: march or jog in place
30 seconds: push-ups
1 minute: march or jog in place
30 seconds: alternating side lunge
1 minute: march or jog in place
30 seconds: side plank reversals
1 minute: march or jog in place
30 seconds: squat jumps

Check heart rate for thirty seconds and multiply by two and take a five-minute walk with light stretching.

With the cooldown, this entire routine is about twenty-one minutes. A PACE routine is not designed to be long but rather very time-efficient. It can be done on alternate days of other types of workouts. For those who have many time constraints, it may be the only workout you do for two or more days per week. Pictures of the thirty-second exercises can be seen below:

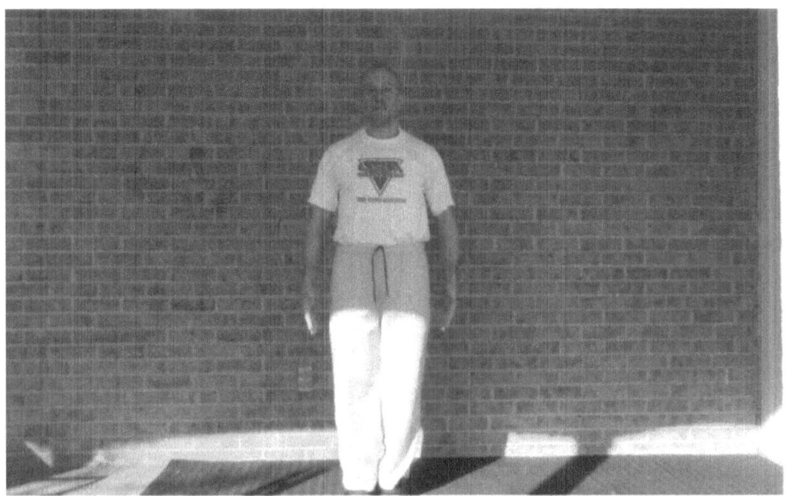

The first movement pattern in this series is the regular jumping jack. It begins in a standing position as seen above. Everyone should remember this one from physical education classes.

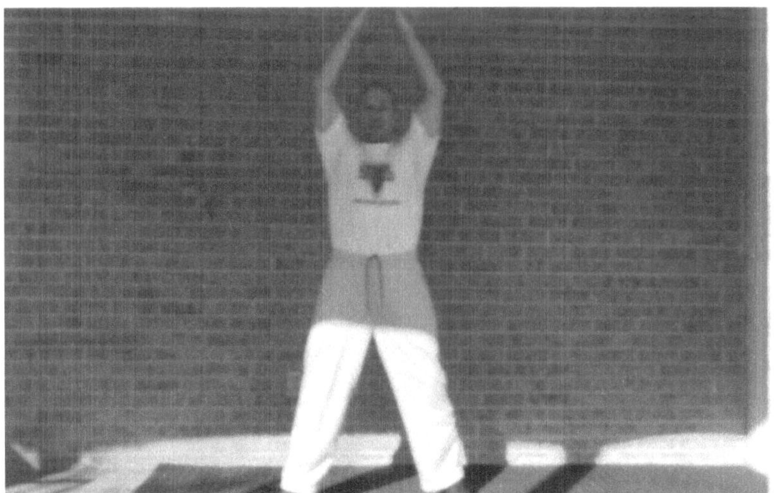

The arms then move overhead and touch while the legs jump out to the side. This can also be referred to as an exercise in the frontal plane.

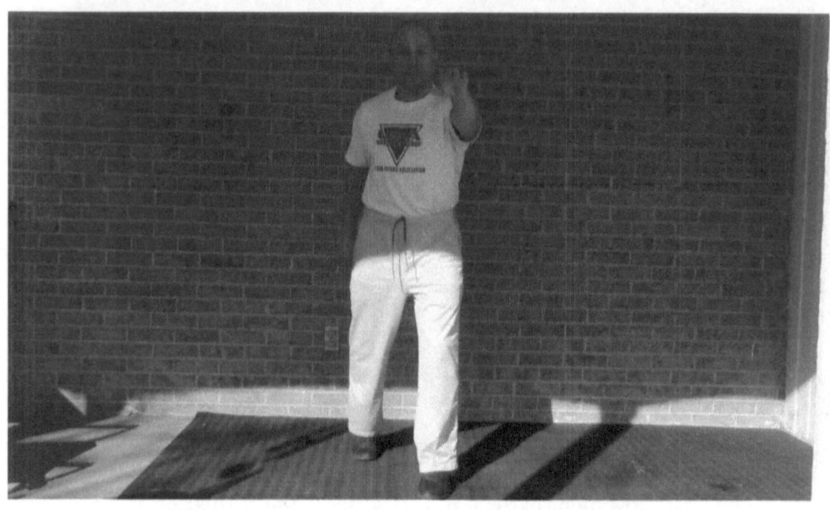

Next, we have the sagittal jack. This exercise can begin with left arm and foot out in front in a staggered position or with the same starting position as the traditional jumping jack.

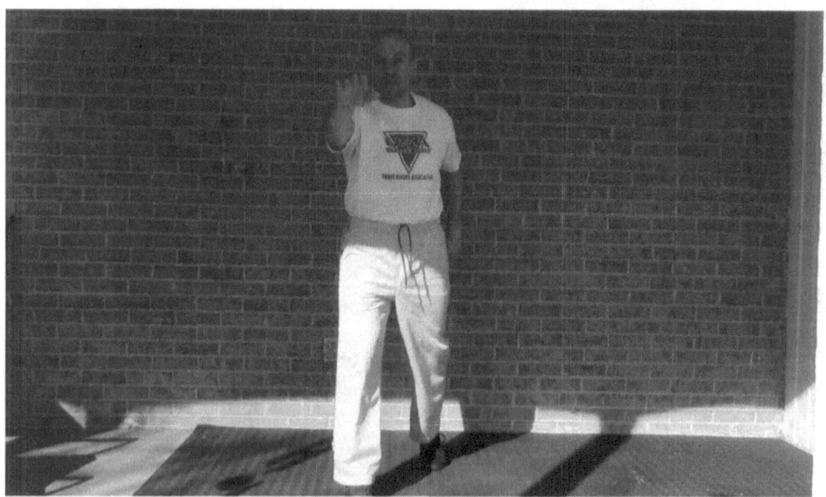

The arms and legs then alternate back and forth.

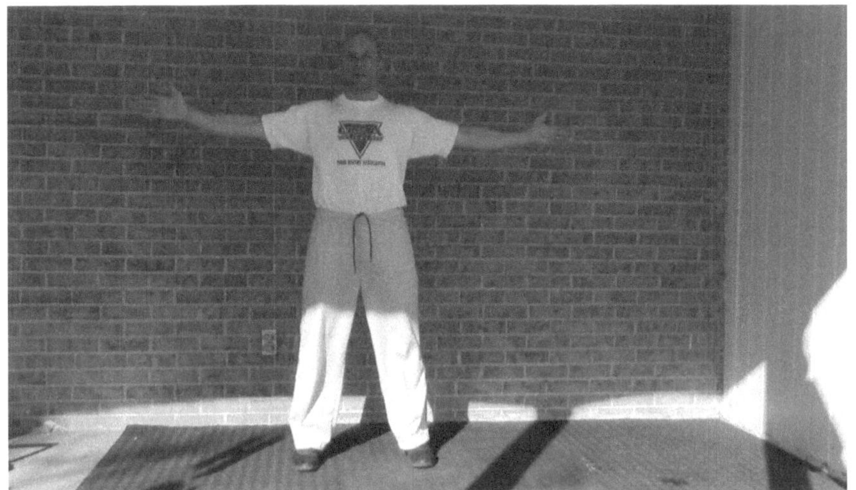

Pictured above is the start of the transverse jack.

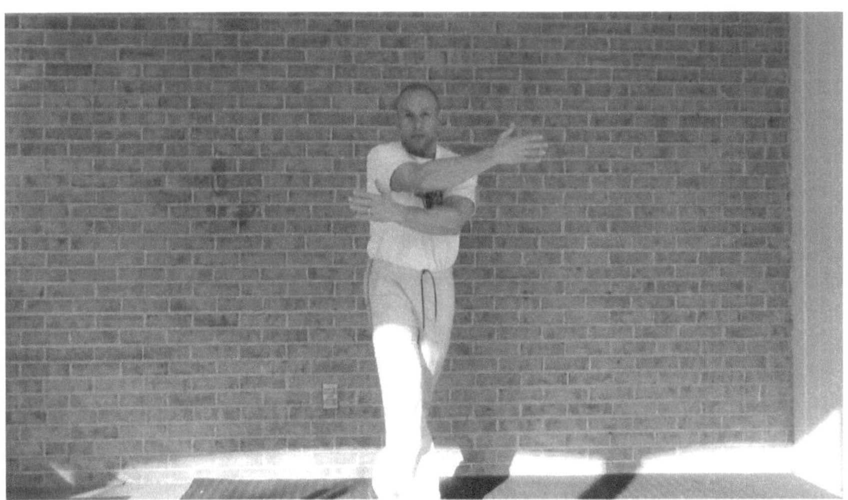

Notice the action of this exercise. The right foot crosses in
front of the left as the left crosses behind. The right arm is also
crossing above the left, and the left arm crosses below.

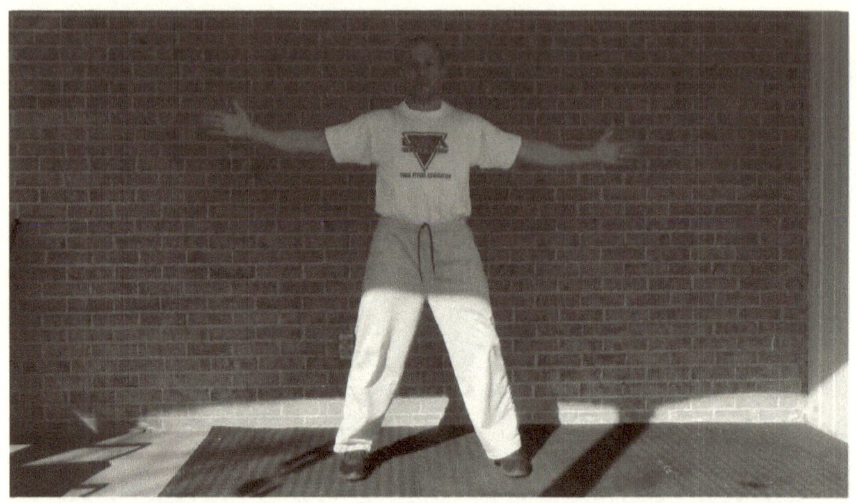

The arms and legs then return to the starting position.

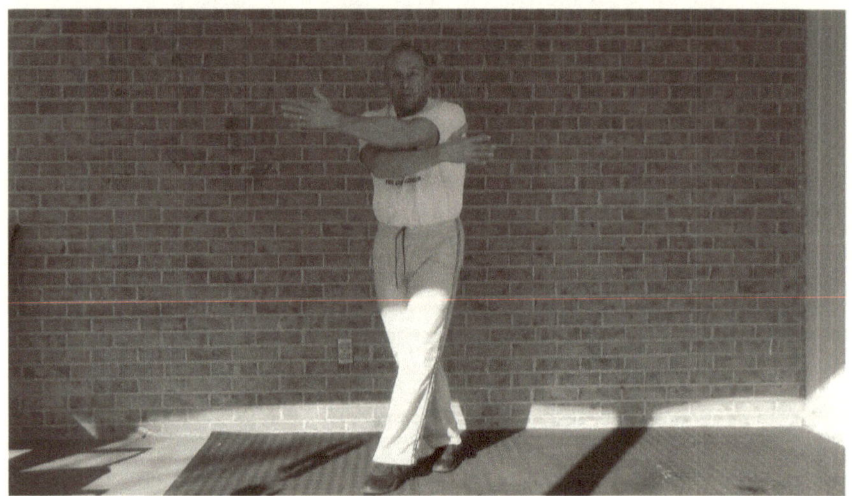

Then the opposite arm and leg have their turn to cross in front,
and the transverse jack continues in this alternating fashion.

Note: all the jack exercises are done with a spring or bounce in the feet for the entire thirty seconds. Of course, modify with a stepping action if needed.

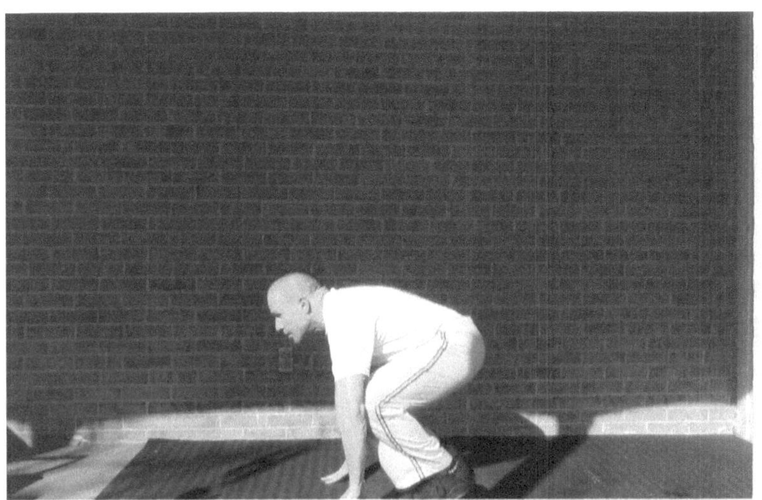

The classic burpee begins in a standing position and then goes to a crouched position with hands touching the floor as shown above.

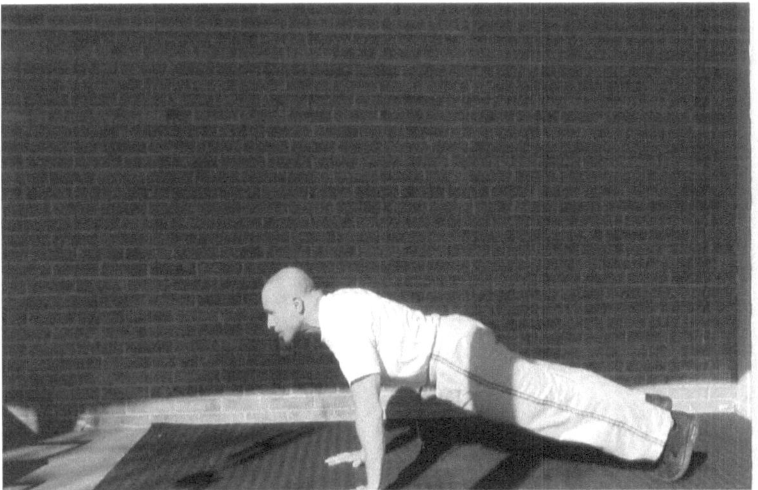

The legs then kick back, and the participant goes into a plank. At this point, a push-up is optional.

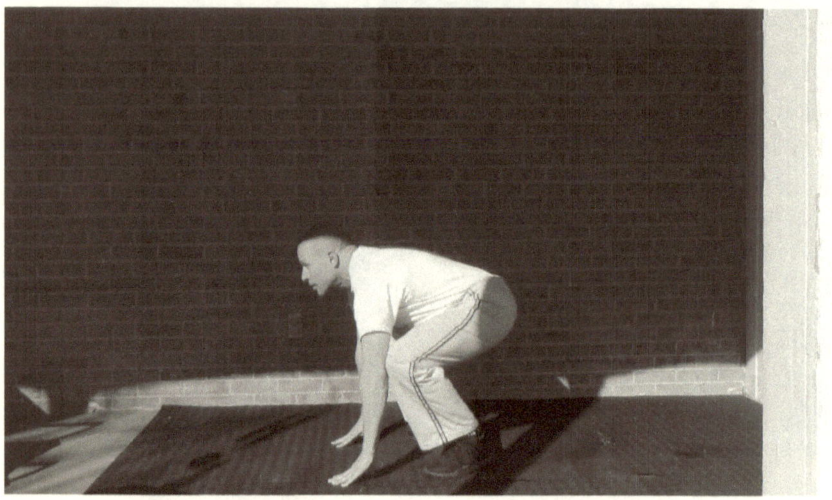

Here, the legs jump back into the crouched position.

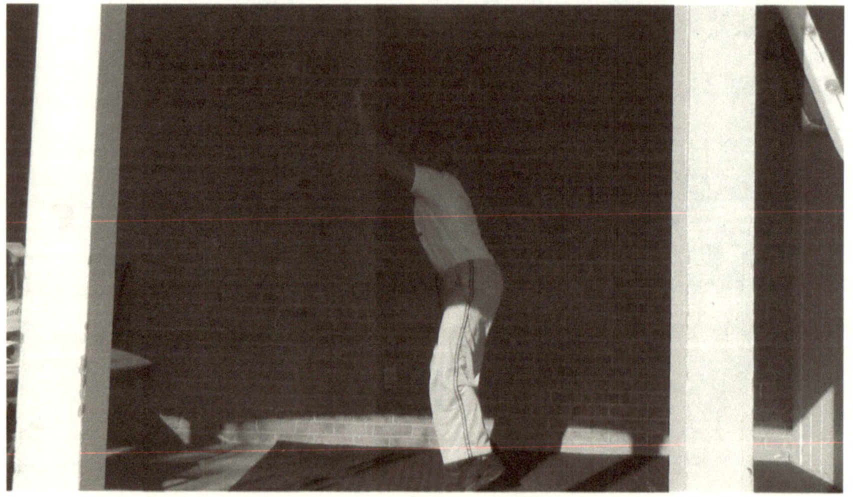

A jump then occurs with arms extended.

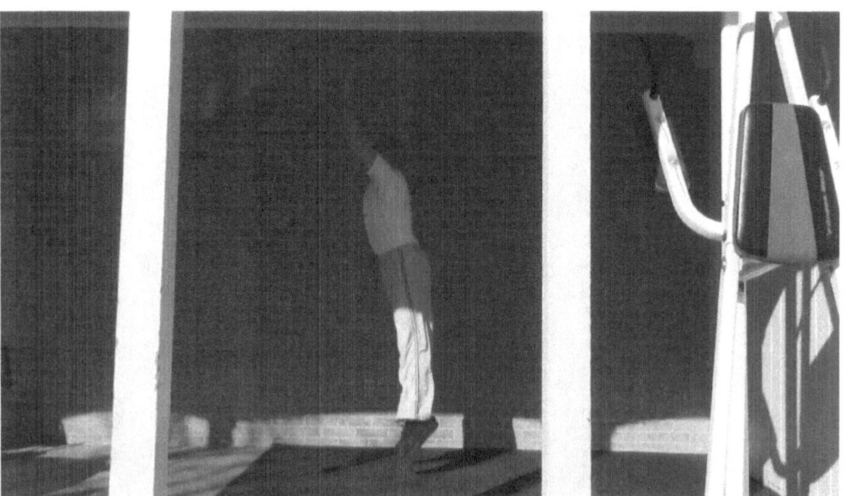

Above the participant is jumping into full extension. Following the jump, you land back into the crouched position and continue.

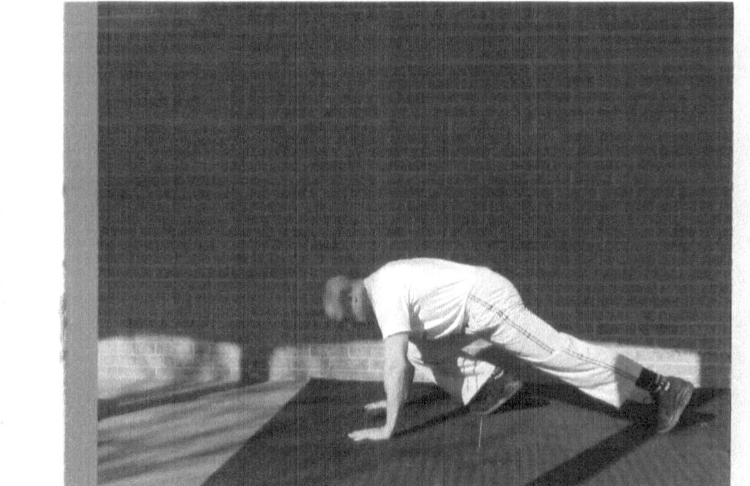

Another classic calisthenics exercise is the mountain climber. It may begin in a plank position or in the position seen above with staggered foot position.

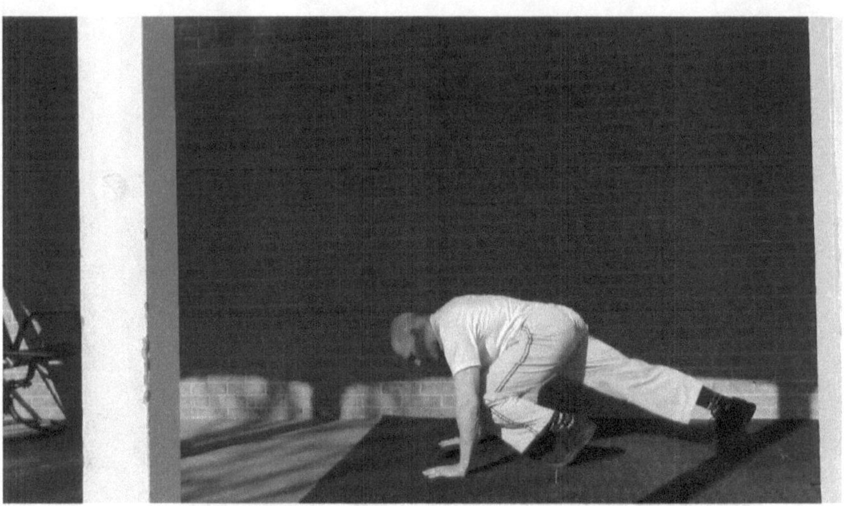

As the shoulders remain stable, the legs alternate a
powerful flexion and extension pattern.

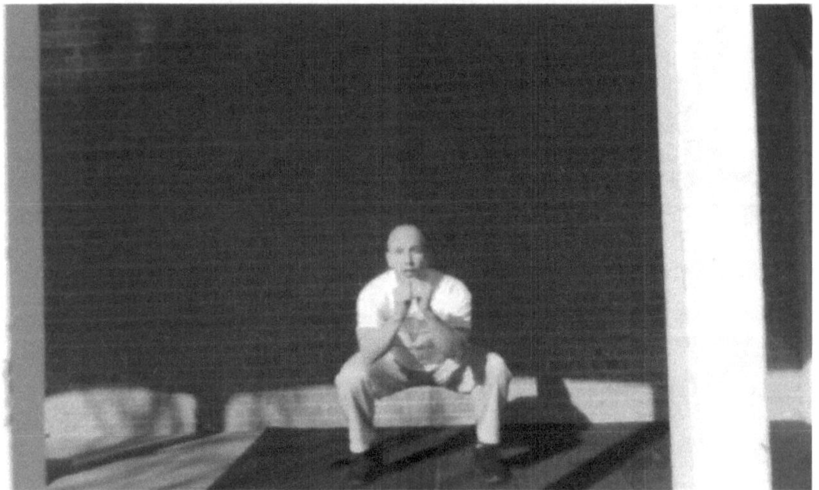

Body weight squats are done to as low a position as reasonably possible.

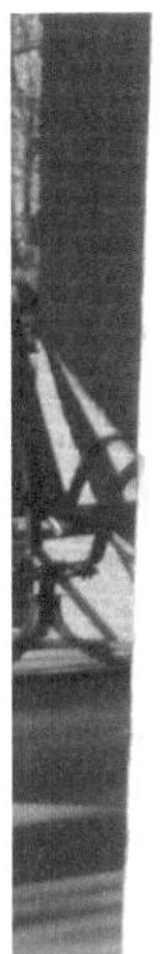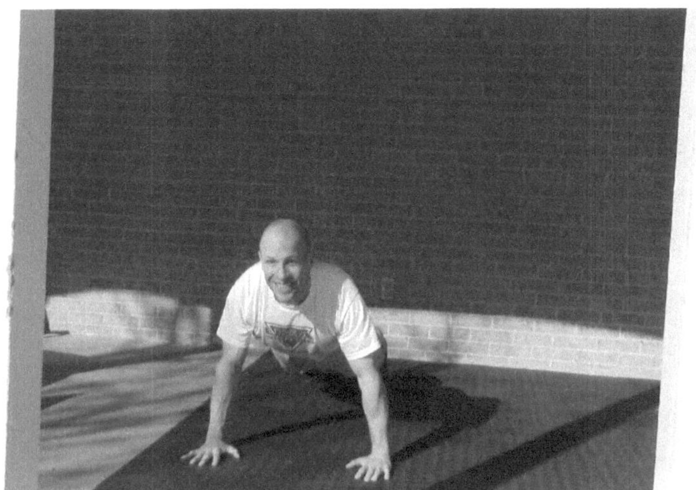

Push-ups are started with proper position as seen above.

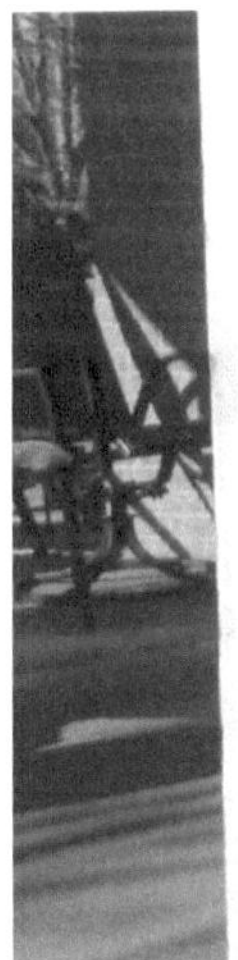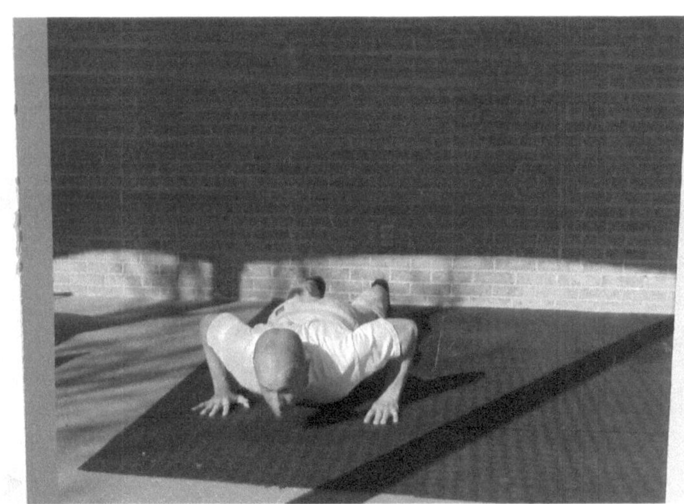

The down movement should have eye elbows go to at least ninety degrees as the rest of the body remains in a straight line.

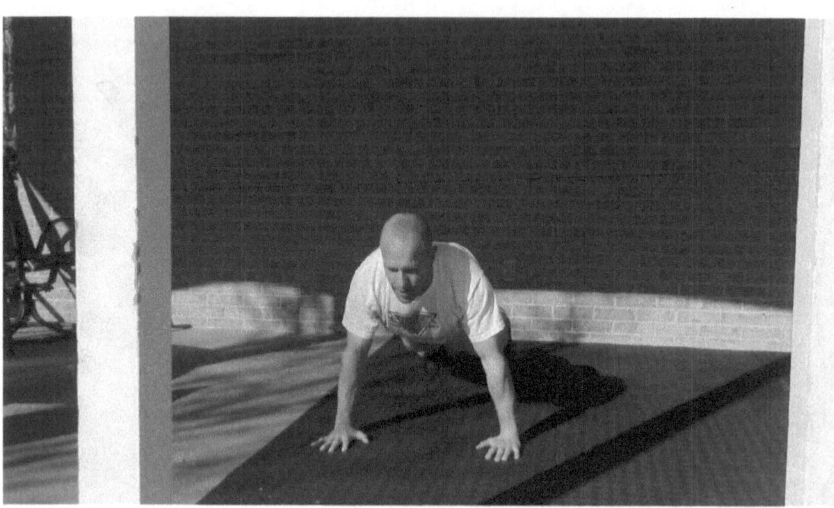

Full extension at the arms completes the repetition along with proper alignment through the body.

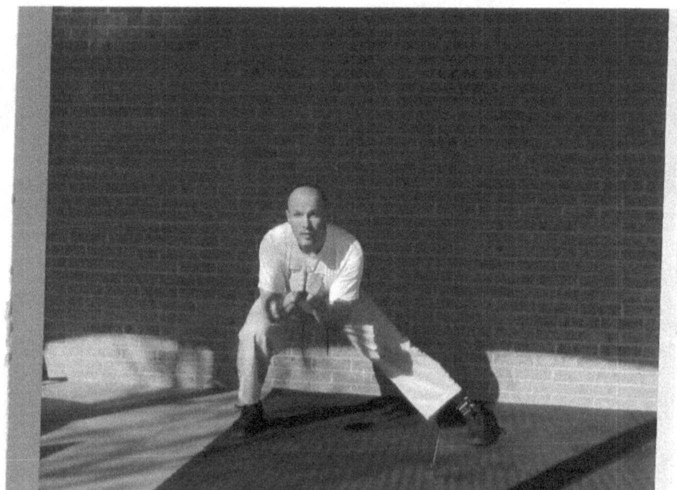

Alternating side lunge starts in a natural standing position. A side luge then occurs with feet pointing straight ahead.

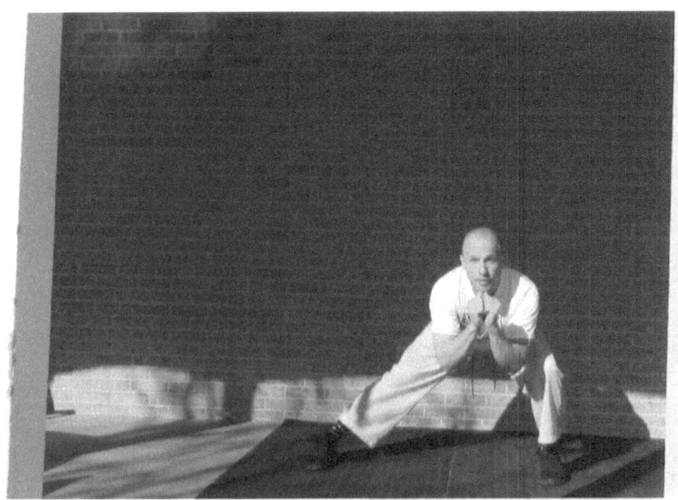

A return to the starting position is performed and
then a side lunge to the other side.

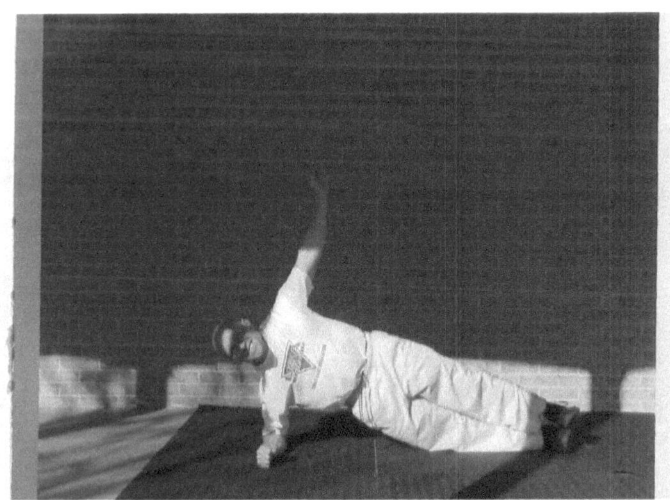

Side plank reversals start in a side plank position
with load-bearing joints in alignment.

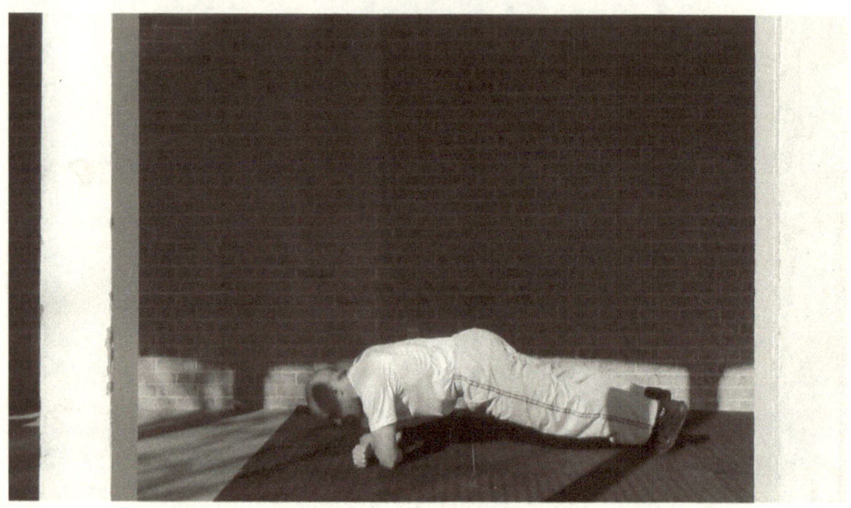

The arm that was up comes down underneath the
body, so a full reversal of position occurs.

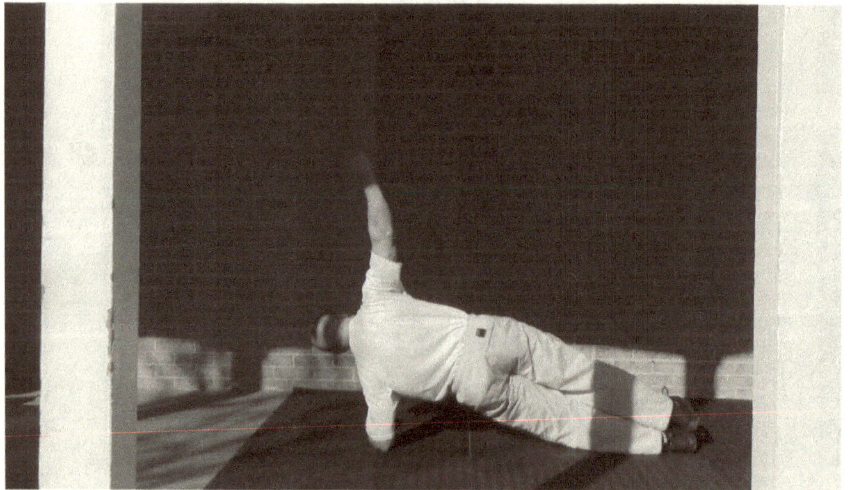

The photo above shows the completion of one side plank reversal.

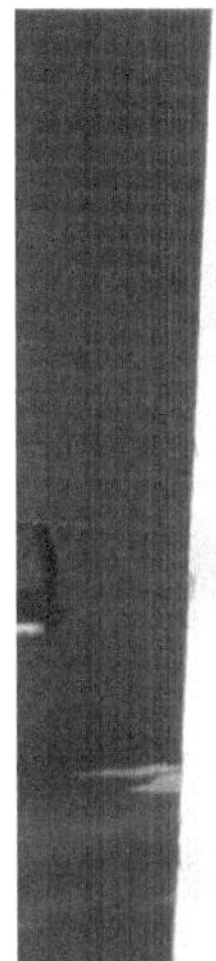
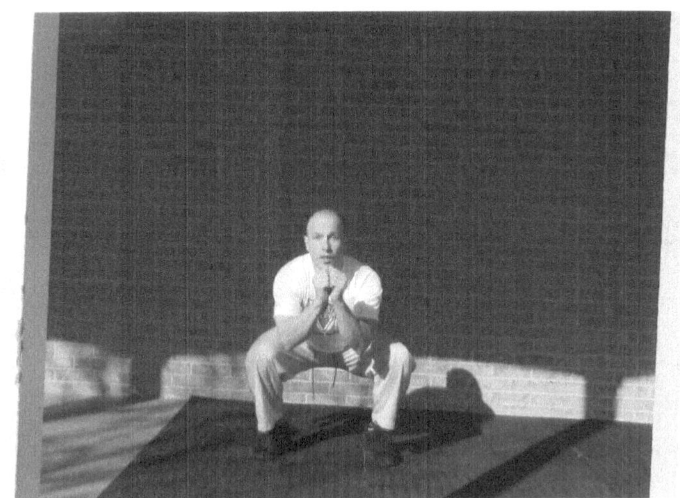

Squat jumps begin like a traditional body weight squat, but an explosive jump occurs on the way out of the squat.

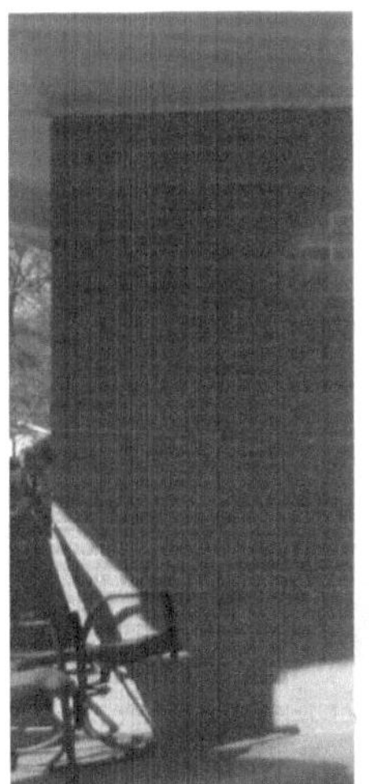
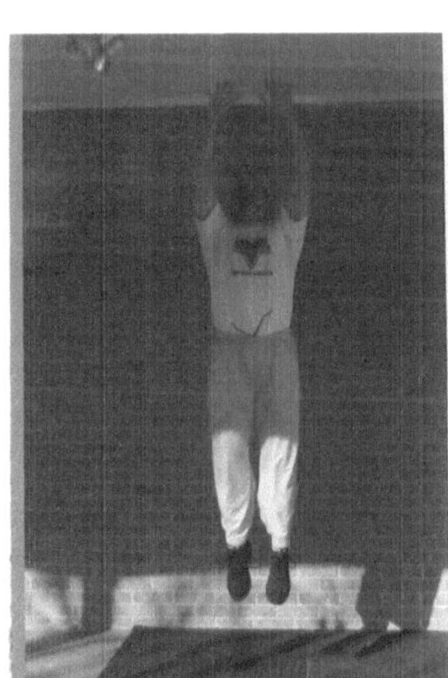
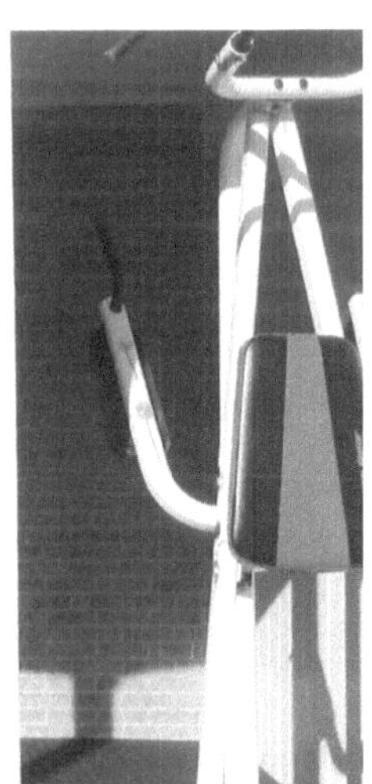

This photo illustrates the explosive jump out of the squat with body fully extended.

Circuit training can manifest through a variety of movements. Some authors have only associated circuit training with weight training or weight training machines. This truly limits the creative approach that can be taken with circuit training. This may also limit the enhancement and conditioning of the heart. Another possible circuit could have this interesting approach:

Push-ups × 25

Pull-ups × 10

Body weight squat × 20

StairMaster × 7 minutes

Note: with the StairMaster, aim for an intensity of 6 to 8 on a scale of 1 to 10. If using a heart rate monitor, strive for your target heart rate zone for that day or a heart rate elevation that is reasonably challenging but not necessarily overwhelming.

The mini circuit above can be done for several rounds. At the completion of the StairMaster, you can take a one- to two-minute rest and go through the circuit several more times. I want you to notice something specific about the circuit though. Take special note of the exercises. You have a push movement (push-up) and a pull movement (pull-up, a squat, which is a lower-body exercise). This is a great approach for muscle balance throughout the body. Following these exercises is the StairMaster. This exercise is done for seven minutes, so it provides aerobic endurance to the circuit.

This circuit does not have to repeat itself. It can lead into something more intricate and challenging. It can be one segment in a much larger circuit. After the StairMaster, for instance, you can go to a dumbbell bench press or a machine chest exercise. This could be followed by a pulling exercise such as a bent-over row or a seated row machine. Notice the push/pull combination forming again with this next group of exercises. This could then be followed by a leg press or calf raise—a lower-body exercise. For our endurance exercise, we could hit the treadmill for five minutes. A third or even a fourth group could follow—all with a push/pull combination, lower-body exercise, and then another aerobic exercise like a stationary bike or elliptical.

Remain mindful that the aerobic exercises in this circuit are for three to seven minutes only. That is long enough. The circuit is designed for muscular strength, muscular endurance, and cardiorespiratory conditioning and endurance. You want to have the time to mix all these in and to do them in an effective manner. Depending on your conditioning level, the StairMaster, treadmill, and others can be done in all energy systems—oxidative, glycolytic, and creatine/phosphate. The oxidative system will engage slow-twitch muscle fibers. The glycolytic energy system will engage both slow- and fast-twitch fibers, and the creatine/phosphate system will engage fast-twitch fibers. In order to tap into different energy systems, various speeds and intensities must be used. This is a wonderful thing because to build the best and most well-rounded body, you should stimulate and engage all muscle fiber types.

Other Fun Challenges for a Super Heart

An old classic bodybuilding strategy is high-rep barbell squats. This is a great anabolic muscle-building strategy, and it is also incredible for building an elite heart muscle. The energy requirement of the heart is immense—especially as the weight increases. Ideally, you should perform squats to parallel at least. The knees should track with the feet, and the back is always straight. After the completion of each rep, take extra breaths. You will need to.

Push-Up

A classic calisthenic exercise, high-rep push-ups can turn into a cardiorespiratory challenge like no other. These push-ups should be done for a full range of motion. The abdomen should touch the ground at the bottom position. A full-elbow extension should be performed on the way up. Load-bearing joint alignment should be maintained for every rep. I have done push-up sets in this fashion that lasted more than twenty minutes. If you have not experienced this, you will be amazed how the heart is pounding after twenty minutes of push-ups and never losing proper position.

Military, law enforcement, and physical education tests require the elbows get to ninety degrees. This is still a viable exercise, but taking the push-up all the way to the ground and all the way up for fifteen minutes or more is another level of conditioning. Be prepared to be amazed. I have a YouTube channel where I go over both types of challenges—Push-Ups as They Should Be Done with George A. James.

Super Sets

A training approach that has been around for many years, super sets provide a tremendous upgrade in intensity. Super sets are done with back-to-back sets with two different exercises. There is no rest in between. The exercises can be opposing muscle groups or very similar in muscles worked. There can be one weight training exercise and body weight exercise or two weight training exercises. Other possibilities could include a medicine ball or plyometric exercise. Super sets are done for specific repetitions or time frame for several sets. It is only two exercises at a time, so the intensity generally is higher as you go back and forth between the two. Depending on the intensity and duration of the workout, a super set routine can consist of only two exercises, or it can be grouped into several groups of two with a rest interval in between.

CHAPTER 10

Final Words and Points to Remember

I N THE 1960S, a doctor for the military, Kenneth Cooper, began to develop a conditioning program for NASA and the United States Air Force. Dr. Cooper was a strong advocate of endurance training. He very well may have coined the phrase *aerobics* from *aerobic*, which means "with oxygen" or "requiring free oxygen." His emphasis was on improving cardiorespiratory health. To maintain ultimate health and wellness, Cooper believed aerobic exercise done through running, cycling, swimming, cross-country skiing, and walking should be performed consistently and more than any other exercise modality. At this point, Cooper did not hold interval training and weight lifting in high regard.

Although Dr. Cooper started his aerobics programs for NASA and the military, his 1968 book *Aerobics* began to influence the entire United States. In the early 1960s, a Gallup poll revealed about 24 percent of Americans were consistent exercisers. At the end of that decade, the number climbed to 50 percent. Dr. Cooper revealed to the *New York Times* in an interview that his emphasis on aerobic training had influenced the country to exercise. His reach continued into the 1970s. He opened the Cooper Institute for Aerobics Research in Texas. Shortly after this, another project began—the Cooper Aerobics Center. It was a fitness center, but in time, it would also include a hotel and spa that attracted high society, including a former president.

Throughout the 1970s, the notoriety of Dr. Cooper increased. He was given credit for enhancing the training of the 1970 Brazilian World Cup championship team. His books on aerobic training were translated into forty-one languages. It appeared that the training approach Dr. Cooper advocated was being thought of as a form of preventive medicine.

Research and Philosophy Continue

Data from Dr. Cooper and his team were adding up. The data and anecdotal evidence pointed to stress relief, vitality, virility, and a long healthy life due to aerobic training. Other studies created a link between fitness and reduced risk factors to the heart. A study by the Cooper Institute was published by the *Journal of the American Medical Association (JAMA)*. Over thirteen thousand people were involved. This study determined that the fitter and more active individuals were not as prone to heart disease and cancer. The study, however, did not consider lifestyle choices like smoking and those who might have health abnormalities.

Eventually, Dr. Cooper would author three other books besides his first that came out in 1968. The four books combined reached more than ten million in sales. The influence and ideas of Cooper continued into the 1970s and 1980s. Other notable names of running and endurance training followed suit with Dr. Cooper—Jim Fixx, Dr. George Sheehan, and Brian Maxwell.

The aerobics movement continued to surge. Another area of endurance training was aerobic dance. This became especially popular for many women. Jane Fonda became one of the key figures in promoting this genre as well as Richard Simmons. Their videos and group classes promoted long-duration activity done primarily at a steady-state pace (sustainable for an hour or longer). Their interesting attire, spandex, leotards, and leg warmers also caught on and became an exercise staple for many.

Today, two decades into the twenty-first century, the concepts developed by Cooper and others are deep within the human psyche. People regularly compartmentalize exercise. They say and were taught that to get any benefit for the cardiovascular system, we must do long-duration activity at a steady state. Weight lifting is a completely separate category that has other benefits, but it is very different from distance running, flexibility training, and plyometrics, just to name a few. What we should realize is that all movement overlaps into other areas of fitness. Movement and strength are synonymous with each other. Any movement performed requires some semblance of strength. We cannot do anything without engaging the cardiovascular/cardiorespiratory system. To simply state cardio training is an entirely separate category of fitness is a statement that is grotesquely misconstrued.

Once upon a time, the American population had few avid runners out in the streets and parks. Today, the number is about 65 million who lace up their running shoes and take to the pavement, tracks, or trails. Before the pandemic of 2020, exercise classes like Zumba, Step Aerobics, and an assortment of others were generally packed with participants. The majority are in search of their aerobic exercise. This is the mentality that has been ingrained for nearly five decades. Since 1968, how far have we come with our aerobic exercise fixation? What exactly is the truth regarding long-duration exercise? What have we learned for certain? The Cooper Institute did much of the early research in the 1960s. Their intentions may have been very good, but they had strong biases toward the exercise style they promoted.

Today, in the United States, things do not look promising. Statistics from the Centers of Disease Control and Prevention illustrate an unhealthy population. More than 60 percent of adults are overweight, and more than 30 percent are at obese levels. Obesity is a key reason why nearly 365,000 lives perish each year. Only smoking surpasses obesity and inactivity as a behavioral cause of death. Heart disease is far greater with 600,000 lives lost yearly. With tens of millions of Americans performing endurance activities, what has gone wrong? Aerobic endurance is supposed to build an impregnable heart, right? What about obesity? The journal *Obesity* revealed in a 2007 study an eye-opening finding. It did point out weight loss benefits with sixty-minute aerobic endurance sessions done for six days per week for a year. (Not all participants exercised this much, but those who did at least 4.2 hours a week for the course of the year actually saw some sort of results.) The women in the study lost an average of five pounds and about a half inch off their waists. The results for the men were better but not by much. The average for the male group was 6.5 pounds, and a little over an inch on their waistlines was lost. Take special note that this study was conducted over a year. The primary exercise was an aerobic form done for an hour most days of the week at moderate to higher levels of intensity. These results are meager. Other forms of exercise or training were not considered.

A 2008 study by the *International Journal of Obesity* had thirty-five overweight and obese men and women. The duration was over twelve weeks. These were sedentary individuals who had the choice of step machines, rowing machines, indoor bikes, or treadmills for their workouts. On average, slightly more than eight pounds was lost in this group. It is also worth mentioning that upon examining the study more closely, it was determined that the heavier individuals were distorting the average. Some of the lighter men and women lost less than expected, and several gained weight. Interestingly, Dr. Cooper touted aerobic exercise for health, longevity, and as a possible preventive measure against heart attacks but not as an answer for weight loss.

Back in Time Once Again

It is true that all forms of exercise may have positive effects on the human organism. As always, though, there are other facts that should be examined and understood. There is another interesting aspect to consider from the aerobics movement. At the beginning, Kenneth Cooper promoted aerobic endurance training, and he believed if you can do more, then do it. His favorite form of exercise was running. He believed it to be the best form of exercise because of its simplicity—all you need is a good pair of running shoes. Cooper was quite fond of elite distance athletes and aerobic enthusiasts who would go the extra miles and minutes. An idea was conveyed that running can be done for your entire life. With running, life would be long, healthy, and good. Simultaneous to this, a different paradigm was growing through the years. It was not as popular—at least not at first.

The *British Journal of Sports Medicine* published insightful but alarming research in 2007. Avid runners were getting injuries—often. Primarily, these were lower leg injuries for runners who did high mileage and had a previous injury. The knees were the most injured area, accounting for 42 percent. Foot and ankles account for 16.9 percent of running injuries. Other injured areas included the Achilles, calf, lower back, and even the hip/pelvic region. Of course, injuries are a part of all sports and exercise activities. The key point here is that if all you do is run long distance, it may turn out to be a hazardous activity. Also, when Dr. Cooper started his aerobics movement, he believed the more, the better. That certainly is not always true. Harvard professor Irene Davis can attest to this. Her observations included 249 recreational runners—all women. They were monitored for a two-year period and had a mileage load of at least twenty miles a week. During this period, 105 of the 249 women did not sustain an injury. Of the 105, only 21 admitted to never sustaining a running injury.

Dr. Cooper believed running was a means to stay youthful, but consistent injuries are a sure way to enhance the aging process. The studies mentioned above demonstrate an unfortunate truth about the prevalence of running injuries. The purpose is not to shun running. Again, all exercise has benefit. The purpose here is to strike a balance with this realization. There are a plethora of reasons why people get hurt and injure themselves. Yes, overuse injuries are one reason. There may also be a lack of recovery for the body. The further the human organism is pushed to its limits, the more rest and nutrition must play a critical role. Alignment is yet something else to consider. Load-bearing joints, ankles, knees, hips, and shoulders play a role in injuries too. The alignment of these joints is necessary for efficient and pain-free movement. Misalignment can occur for nearly anyone with the stress of life and sporting activities. Prolonged sitting at work or traveling also poses problems by shortening muscles. Shortened muscles with misaligned joints added to stressful exercise can pose a painful problem for anyone.

Running and the Heart

Long before Kenneth Cooper, Pheidippides of ancient Greece ran for two days in 490 BC. He arrived back in Athens to report of the Greek victory over the Persians and then dropped dead. This is a legend, but sometimes legends are harbingers for future events. There was a notion that persisted that running was a means to ultimate health and longevity. This idea persisted for many years. One aerobics book that came out in the early 1980s had this quote, "Some thirty million Americans are running religiously, to save their lives—in essence, the quality of life itself." In 1984, the body of Jim Fixx was found on a side of a road in Vermont. Fixx was a long-distance running icon to many and author of *The Complete Book of Running*. He died of a heart attack while running at age fifty-two. An autopsy revealed he had arteriosclerosis, and he had blockage in three arteries of 95 percent, 85 percent, and 50 percent.

Brian Maxwell, who was the creator of PowerBar, was once one of the top marathon runners on earth. He also succumbed to a heart attack at fifty-one. A simple internet search reveals a vast number of marathon runners who have died because of heart abnormalities. Chris McDougall's book *Born to Run* speaks of a legendary ultrarunner, Micah True. He surprisingly passed away of cardiac arrhythmia while running on a trail in New Mexico at fifty-eight. Avid jogger Miles Frost passed away while out for a jog. He had an unknown heart abnormality. He was only thirty-one. His father was Sir David Frost, a British broadcaster who died of a heart attack two years earlier.

Are the examples above genetic abnormalities? Jim Fixx lived to be fifty-two. His father only lived to be forty-three. He outlived his dad by nine years. Maybe the running prolonged his life. This may be true to some extent. Physical activities and exercise of all types have proven to be beneficial. Throughout the 1950s and

1960s, various studies demonstrated a greater correlation with coronary heart disease and sedentary jobs as compared to more active positions. *The Lancet*, a British medical journal, was one such source where these types of studies were being reported. It reported the death rate of bus drivers to bus conductors from coronary heart disease in middle age. The bus conductors who were much more active on their jobs had a smaller death rate than the drivers who were sitting for many hours on their job. These studies continued. In 1975, the *New England Journal of Medicine* published a twenty-two-year study with longshoremen in California. More than six thousand men were considered for their type of job. One group loaded and unloaded cargo, and another were administrative workers with much less physical activity. Again, the group with greater physical exertion showed a significant difference with less coronary heart disease.

Take note again that in these examples the difference seemed to be more physical activity. It was not aerobic activity necessarily. Various studies have shown that all exercise or activity promote a vibrant life in a number of ways, and all types of movement can be beneficial. The notion proposed by Cooper and others since the 1960s that aerobic exercise is the most important for heart health and longevity is not necessarily true. In 1984, cardiologist Henry Solomon challenged the ideology of Cooper and others in *The Exercise Myth*. He claimed that passing a fitness test, including a stress test created by Cooper, was not an indication of an absence of ill heart health. Solomon explained something very interesting. A stress test demonstrates exercise performance. Coronary heart disease, on the other hand, is structural. The narrowing of the coronary arteries is not identified through a stress test. Just in the last couple years, a very interesting discovery was made. A Harvard study used firefighters from Indiana who were forty years of age or slightly older. A direct correlation was made with push-ups and cardiovascular health. It was determined that if a man could do forty push-ups or more, there was a 96 percent reduced chance of heart attack, stroke, and heart failure. A cardiologist from Arkansas who reviewed this research admitted that the ability to do push-ups is a better indicator of heart health than a stress test at the doctor's office.

What have we leaned since the late 1960s when the aerobics phenomenon began? Did the aerobics boom create a society that was resistant to heart problems? Heart disease did decrease significantly from the late '60s and into the twenty-first century. In recent years though, the numbers have been stagnant. Can anyone state unequivocally that aerobic training is the reason why? They cannot. Nutrition, stress, and lifestyle may be contributing factors as well. Aerobic training can and probably was a contributing factor for the lowering of heart disease too. It does improve efficiency of the heart and lungs. Be mindful that there is not a single exercise or type of movement pattern that is the epitome of all that fitness is.

Dr. Peter Schnohr, who considered the Copenhagen City Heart study as part of his studies, provided interesting insight into jogging. The study observed the pace, quantity, and frequency of joggers. From his observations, it was determined that light to moderate joggers have a lower mortality rate than a sedentary population. The excessive runners or joggers revealed what might be a surprise to many. This group had a mortality rate that was comparable to the sedentary group. Additional running, perhaps to an excessive amount, did not produce longevity and healthier individuals. Cardiologists James O' Keefe, Peter Schnohr, and Carl Lavie all caution against high amounts of endurance training. This recommendation is especially true for those fifty and over who have greater potential for cardiovascular damage. A key point to realize too is that there is a law of diminishing returns. More is not always better for anything, including exercise.

In 2012, I began working for a company that advocated for high-intensity training as an introductory session for new members. A creative approach was emphasized, and a plethora of various exercises in circuits, super sets, etc. could be used. The idea was to have a potentially new client be in awe of how hard they would train if we were their trainer. Unfortunately, not very much was mentioned about individual differences and lifestyle. I think common sense prevailed in most examples though. High-intensity exercise and programming have played a large role throughout the fitness industry in the last couple of decades. The concept here is to have greater caloric expenditure and reach fitness goals faster. This can be conveyed through small groups, classes, and one-on-one training. Establishments like CrossFit and Orange Theory primarily emphasize higher-intensity training. Higher intensity can mean heavier breathing rate, faster exercise pace, and doing more in a shorter period of time.

Many gyms and training protocols in the past recommended long-duration aerobic training. As a student at Slippery Rock University in the early 2000s, I recall being taught that ideally everyone should have at least thirty minutes of aerobic training for three separate days a week or more. Recent research in exercise physiology has shed light on an interesting phenomenon that challenges this approach. Excess postexercise oxygen consumption is a term that has gained notoriety with short intense workouts. These types of routines may burn the same or more calories than a long monotonous session of an hour or perhaps longer. There are a couple of credible reasons for this. With higher intensity, movement efficiency diminishes. When this happens, greater energy is needed to perform an exercise or workout compared to slower aerobic training. Perhaps more significantly, there is a change in metabolism after the exercise session. After a challenging workout, more oxygen is consumed, and a higher metabolic rate follows. So you are burning more calories even at rest. It is believed that an early morning session induces this response even more.

Many commercial gyms once emphasized the long aerobic activity as a hallmark of a workout for members. Educational institutions did the same. The tide has turned toward brevity and intensity. Even Dr. Cooper changed his perspective on how much aerobic training was best. He once felt that the more mileage, the better. As research evolved, he later stated that fifteen to twenty miles should suffice for positive health achievement. Others argue that this is too much.

Benefits of short workouts like intervals are something that has caught great interest and popularity. Why is this the case? It may be helpful to consider some of these items again. One of the key characteristics is the enhanced metabolic rate, which can be effected much longer after the workout than a long drawn-out aerobic session. Greater caloric expenditure is another hallmark of higher-intensity training. With more calories being burned, ultimately, body composition becomes healthier. Time efficiency is a precious component in our modern era. If your time is very limited, the good news is you do not need a great deal of time. Twenty to thirty minutes will suffice. Effective workouts can be less than twenty minutes too. You should make the time meaningful, however, through greater intensity. As far as creativity and program design, the sky is the limit. There are so many options at your disposal. HIIT, circuit training, and PHA are all separate variations, but each can be altered with different exercises and time elements. Circuit training for instance has an interesting history. In the last two or three decades, many commercial gyms have viewed circuit training as weight training performed on Cybex or Nautilus equipment. Various fitness and strength training authors have written that circuit training is not as beneficial for the heart as aerobic training. The real truth is that circuit training has its origin from the late 1950s. Two British physical educators, Morgan and Adamson, devised circuit training to be a wide assortment of exercises that included weight training, calisthenics, and gymnastics. A routine like this could strengthen the heart far more than an hour on the elliptical, watching ESPN. Most importantly, high-intensity sessions with short duration can be super for the heart. A study on high-intensity interval training demonstrated increased elasticity of arteries and veins. The increased blood volume causes this to happen. Current research also suggests that a HIIT routine may be more tolerable for those with coronary artery disease because of the changing intensity. A long moderate workout is monotonous with the intensity remaining constant.

Should every workout be a brief high-intensity workout? A vast amount of evidence and research indicate positive outcomes from this type of training done consistently. It appears that a very high percentage involved in the fitness industry are now advocating for brief high-intensity episodes as opposed to endurance emphasized physical training. In my experience, I have observed trainers and enthusiasts scoff at the notion of any kind of endurance training—thinking it is a useless waste of time. Is this true? Does steady-state endurance exercise serve any viable purpose? With all research and knowledge, it is wise to take an open-minded and humble approach—especially when it comes to fitness through the eyes of the heart. First, we should consider two aspects of physical training. General physical preparation (GPP) is one, and the other is specific physical preparation (SPP). As the name indicates, GPP is general fitness. It should consist of a variety of exercises to broaden the scope of physical development. This is good because we have type I, type IIA, and type IIB muscle fibers, and to build the most resilient body, all fibers should be exercised. GPP may consist of endurance work with a bike or swim, body weight calisthenics, various agility drills for sports, and super setting resistance exercises. SPP is an advanced form of training. It does not always have to be more intense than GPP. There are other variables like the level of athlete or participant and where someone is in their training cycle. SPP considers a particular sport of fitness goal or the training law of specificity. SPP examples include a track athlete performing intervals to have a greater fitness base for their event. It could also be an Olympic weight lifter doing two sessions a day—an explosive one and a strength-focused training period. Of course, an endurance athlete could be an example too. Obviously, long-duration training will be needed for a distance runner, swimmer, rower, or cyclist. Realize though that an elite distance athlete is far greater than the average gym member on a stationary bike, so much of their training will be greater than a simple steady-state training pattern. The main point is that SPP is a singular focus with some variation that supports the ultimate goal.

So in consideration of GPP and SPP, more or less endurance work may be required as an athlete or fitness participant evolves with changing goals and requirements. An athlete who has been focusing on SPP for a while may go back to GPP after a competition season has ended. This may prevent overuse injuries and allow a refocus on other fitness attributes to make for a well-rounded and fit individual. Endurance/aerobic training will probably fit in to this plan somewhere. Endurance training will always have a place in health and fitness, but it is not the end all and be all of health and fitness that some have tried to make it into.

A Lesson to Remember

Finally, an important lesson should always be remembered. Think of this possible scenario that I have witnessed on more than one occasion in the fitness industry. An overweight individual comes into the gym to meet with their trainer. The trainer believes they know the right approach for their chubby client. The client is looking for success after not being able to reach their goals for the past five years. The trainer has bought into the brief workout with high intensity for greater caloric expenditure. They train together for weeks and then months for two, three, and sometimes four sessions a week. Homework is given also to supplement the training sessions they do together. The workouts are tough, and the client does his best. As time elapses, the body composition of the client does not change. Sometimes, workouts are missed due to nagging injuries and occasional colds. On top of this, progress has waned. The client has even gotten fatter. What is the problem?

The trainer has neglected a golden principle—a catabolic state plus a catabolic state does not equal an anabolic state. It never has and never. It does not matter if you're twenty, fifty, or seventy-five years of age. It does not matter who you are or who you think you are. The principle rings true for the lifetime of any person. When the client and trainer were first getting to know each other, the client expressed that their lifestyle was very busy. The nutritional approach was not consistent, and often the client would get three hours of sleep at night at best. Despite these weak attributes, the client would religiously meet with his trainer the next day after inadequate nutrition and little sleep. He would train hard, break into profuse sweating, while his heart pumped furiously. The lifestyle and training did not correlate. The client did not understand that everything that happens in the gym has to be accounted for outside the gym. Unfortunately, his trainer did not understand this either.

Physical training alone is not enough. Training includes lifestyle, intelligence, proper planning, rest, positive mental attitude, and sound nutrition. The best workouts are only as good as everything else that is happening in an individual's life. The client in the example above needed to focus on a balanced lifestyle. They needed to get back to appropriate sleep cycles so their hormones could heal them at night and help build muscle and recovery.

High-intensity training was not appropriate for the example above. You see the client was not able to recover from very intense workouts. He needed to gradually evolve into higher intensity as important lifestyle changes were made along the way. Cortisol levels were elevated too often. This caused additional unwanted weight gain. In this example, those short intense workouts that are supposed to be so great for the heart and metabolism completely backfired. In order to push the body hard, with sweat unloading down the forehead and a heart that will not surrender, you have to earn it. It is earned with a balanced life that is conducive to hard training. The client needed to do light aerobic activity, alignment and breathing exercises, body weight movements, and core development at a reasonable pace for their lifestyle. Doing intense circuits, super sets, and intervals took too much energy the client could not replenish because of a poor overall lifestyle. All exercise is good and has its place, but it should always coincide with fitness goals and ambitions and the energy you have and are truly willing to give. Exercise must be nourished with what you do before and after the workout. This is a powerful lesson the heart and body will always recognize.

APPENDIX A

T HIS SECTION PROVIDES additional exercise ideas and combinations to build a strong heart and body. It can be helpful in igniting other thoughts for circuits and super set routines.

Mini Circuits

Group 1

1) Plyometric push-ups
2) Alternating dumbbell row in push-up position
3) Bench jumps

Group 2

1) Cable exchanging press (each arm is moving simultaneously as press is performed with cable machine)
2) Cable exchanging prone row (each arm is moving simultaneously as row is performed with cable)
3) Cable duck under (have a partner hold cable and duck under back and forth without hitting cable and using a height that is challenging)

<u>**Group 3**</u>

1) Alternating reverse lunge
2) Two-hand kettlebell push press
3) Pull-up

<u>**Group 4**</u>

1) Goblet squat on BOSU
2) Kettlebell swing with two hands
3) Dips

<u>**Group 5**</u>

1) Barbell high pull (clean or snatch grip)
2) One-arm dumbbell bench press
3) Split squat (body weight or with dumbbell, kettlebell, or barbell)

Super Sets:

<u>**Group 1**</u>

1) Barbell front squat
2) Kettlebell power clean

<u>**Group 2**</u>

1) Medicine ball slams
2) Jump squat

<u>**Group 3**</u>

1) Medicine ball slams with rotation
2) Jumping jacks

<u>**Group 4**</u>

1) Push-up
2) Jump rope

<u>**Group 5**</u>

1) Burpee with push-up
2) Box on heavy bag

Well, as for the sets, reps, time, and intensity, that is up to your heart.

APPENDIX B

References

Baechle, Thomas R., and Earle, Roger W., eds. 2000. *Essentials of Strength Training and Conditioning*, second edition. National Strength and Conditioning Association. Champaign, Illinois: Human Kinetics.

McArdle, William D., Katch, Frank I., and Katch, Victor L. 2000. *Essentials of Exercise Physiology*, second edition. Philadelphia, Baltimore, New York, London, Buenos Aires, Hong Kong, Sydney, Tokyo: Lippincott, Williams, and Wilkins.

Brooks, Douglas S. 1997. *Program Design for Personal Trainers*. Human Kinetics. Champaign, Illinois.

Sears, Al, MD. 2004. *The Doctor's Heart Cure*. St. Paul, Minnesota: Dragon Door Publications.

Jones, Brian. 2006. *The Conditioning Handbook*. Nevada City, California: Ironmind Enterprises.

Pert, Candace. 1997. *Molecules of Emotion*. New York, New York: Simon and Schuster/Scribner.

Yehoshua Zohar. March 2012. Milo. *The Pros and Cons of Circuit Training*. Nevada City, California: Ironmind Enterprises.

Childre, Doc, Martin, Howard, and Beech, Donna. 1999. *The Heartmath Solution*. New York, New York: Harper Collins.

Godwin, Jeff. 1988. *Dancing with Demons*. Chino, California: Chick Publications.

Ballantyne, Craig, and Ratcliff, Chelsea. 2017. *The Great Cardio Myth*. Beverly, Massachusetts: Fairwinds.

Burke, Edmund R., ed. 1998. *Precision Heart Rate Training*. Champaign, Illinois: Human Kinetics.

APPENDIX C

Statin-Lowering Cholesterol Drugs
Atorvastatin (Lipitor)
Fluvastatin (Lescol, Lescol XL)
Lovastatin (Mevacor, Altoprev)
Pravastatin (Pravachol)
Rosuvastatin (Crestor)
Simvastatin (Zocor)
Pitavastatin (Livalo)

Side Effects of Statins

*headache
*nausea
*vomiting
*constipation
*diarrhea
*rash

*weakness
*muscle pain
*liver failure
*rhabdomyolysis (death/injury of muscle tissue)

www.ingramcontent.com/pod-product-compliance
Lightning Source LLC
Chambersburg PA
CBHW051456250726
48655CB00001B/445

9 781664 110410